Born
Beautiful

Born Beautiful

The African American Teenager's Complete Beauty Guide

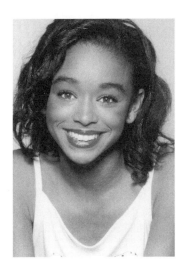

Alfred Fornay

AN AMBER BOOK

John Wiley & Sons, Inc.

Published by John Wiley & Sons, Inc., New York
Published simultaneously in Canada

Produced by Amber Books Publishing, 1334 East Chandler Boulevard, Suite 5-b67, Phoenix, AZ 85048

Design and production by Navta Associates, Inc.

This publication is designed to provide accurate and authoritative information in regard to the subject matter covered. It is sold with the understanding that the publisher is not engaged in rendering professional services. If professional advice or other expert assistance is required, the services of a competent professional person should be sought.

ISBN: 0-471-40275-3

Printed in the United States of America
10 9 8 7 6 5

To all teenagers discovering their own sense of style

My grandnieces,
Tayler, Alexis, Maryah, Caelyn, Crystal,
Alyssa, Kelly, Kayle, and Kenya

And their parents and aunt,
Sharry, Sharmyn, Carla, Darla, and Troy

CONTENTS

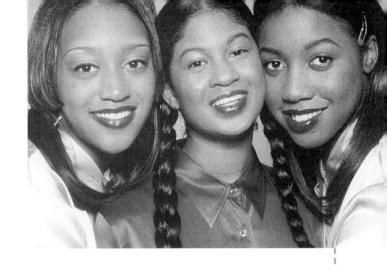

Foreword by Cynthia Horner   ix

Introduction   1

CHAPTER 1
Beautiful Skin   3

Skin Science 101   4

Your Natural Protection   5

Your True Skin   6

What's the Sun Got to Do with It?   13

Your Skin Type   16

CHAPTER 2
The Basics of a Flawless Complexion   23

Love Your Skin   23

The Oily Skin Regimen   30

The Dry Skin Regimen   35

The Combination (Normal) Skin Regimen   39

The Sensitive Skin Regimen   42

Skin Problems   46

Love Your Facial Skin Color   49

Your True Color   52

Create Your Specific Foundation Look   53

Blending Your Foundation   54

Placing the Foundation on Your Face   56

Improving the Look of Your Skin   56

Concealers   57

Face Powders   59

CHAPTER 3
The Color Workshop   65

Choosing the Right Colors for Your Best Look   65

Breaking through the Rules   66

Your Undertones   67

The Flair for Color   69

A New Eye on Color   69

Gorgeous Makeup from Day to Date 71

Your Eyes and the Use of Color 73

Eyebrow Grooming   78

Eyeliner Essentials   81

Eye-Catching Eye Shadow   83

Mascara   84

Blushers for a Special Glow   85

Do You Know Your Face Shape?   88

Your Fabulous Lips   90

Let's Review!! The Ultra-Grand Makeup
    Application   96

CHAPTER 4
Those Little Extras That Define You!   101

Smellin' Good—Making Sense of Your
    Fragrance Choices   102

Fragrance in Your Life   104

The Scented Bath   106

Your Glorious Nails—They Can Be Even
    More Beautiful!   108

Nail Care   113

The 411 on Tattoos and Body Piercing
    119

Natural Henna Tattoos   121

Body Piercing   125

CHAPTER 5
Chic Hairstyles and Care for Your Hair   127

How Should I Wear My Hair?   128

Hair Weaves, Braids, and Extensions   132

Natural Styles   133

Straightened Hair   134

Now Let's Do Color!   134

Speaking of Hair!   140

CHAPTER 6
Food, Fashion, and Fitness for a Better You   143

Fast Break   144

Snacks   144

Got a Sweet Tooth?   145

Water   146

Try Vegetarian Nutrition   146

For a Healthy Vegetarian Diet, Variety
    Is the Key   149

What about Protein?   149

Other Important Nutrients   150

Getting Fit with Your Favorite
    Exercises   151

Rest and Relaxation   152

Conclusion: The Last Word on
    Beauty   157

Acknowledgments   159

Index   163

See the Fornay Color Chart in the middle of the book.

FOREWORD

by Cynthia Horner, editor-in-chief,
Right On! magazine

E ver since I was a little girl, I have enjoyed playing with makeup and cosmetics. The whiff of powder on puffs, the glistening tubes of lipstick gleaming from glamorous cases, and the pungent scents of perfumes emanating from my mother's bureau linger in my mind. I read with enthusiasm every pamphlet I could order from cosmetics companies, and eagerly combed through magazines, searching for information on beauty and personal hygiene.

This was many years ago, long before the current magazines that we see on the newsstands or on salon tables ever existed. It was also long before African Americans and other models of color were prominently featured in advertising and editorial spreads. So for me, learning about beauty sort of happened by trial and error. Today's teens don't have that problem.

First and foremost, contemporary recording artists, models and actresses, and athletes are in a position to serve as visible role models. They come in a myriad of shades ranging from ebony to café au lait, wearing bone-straight tresses to easy-to-care-for dreads. And guess what? Through the newfound emphasis of our uniqueness as individuals, today's teens are becoming more confident in their ability to be beautiful, too. However, information addressing the concerns of African American teens has rarely been available in book form until now.

Fortunately, through the publication of *Born Beautiful,* young women (and older ones, too) can tap into author Alfred Fornay's precious knowledge and practical advice. As my fingers turned the pages of this priceless beauty bargain, I discovered beautiful blazing chapters on "Chic Hairstyles and Care for Your Hair," "The Color Workshop," "Food, Fashion, and Fitness for a Better You," "The Basics of a Flawless

Complexion," and "Beautiful Skin." No pertinent topic is ignored, and contemporary trends like body piercings and tattoos make their way into the pages as well. With such an insightful, cleverly written book at their disposal, readers will find that Alfred Fornay's beauty book really makes a whole lot of "scents."

INTRODUCTION

Y ou are a beautiful teenager! You are so wonderful! You were *Born Beautiful!* You are going to have fun learning how to bring out the attractive, appealing person you've dreamed and thought about being.

You'll learn everything you want to know about great skin, gorgeous makeup, chic hairstyles, and more.

You'll see great pictures of Ananda Lewis, Destiny's Child, Brandy, Beyoncé, and Changing Faces, who share their secret beauty tips with you. I will give you the 411 on all the things that you really need to and want to know about: The Basics of a Flawless Complexion, Gorgeous Makeup from Day to Date, Chic Hairstyles and Care for Your Hair, Ten Steps to Fabulous Nails, Choosing the Right Colors for Your Best Look, Food, Fashion, and Fitness for a Better You, Making Sense of Your Fragrance Choices, the 411 on Tattoos and Body Piercing, and other fad favorites.

Teenagers around the globe who observe your style on *Soul Train;* BET's *Teen Summit,* MTV, and VH1, all admire your special talents and abilities, which have been adapted by designers at mainstream fashion houses worldwide, all coming from your individuality and style.

Every teenager has within her exciting potentialities that can be discovered and nurtured to help her become a more attractive, more interesting, more appealing personality. *Born Beautiful* has been designed specifically to help you make the most of that potential, so that you can achieve success and happiness in your schoolwork, social and religious activities, and in your personal life.

The advice of experts from related fields has been brought together in this book to discuss and provide solutions to questions you might have about your complexion, hair, fragrances, and health.

And there's lots of fun stuff, including: FYI (For Your Information), Basic Beauty Facts (little things that you should know about), Reviews (so you'll remember everything), Celebrity Secret Beauty Tips (from your fave celebs), Teen Tips (advice from teens just like you), Quizzes (and of course the answers), Smart and Sensible Suggestions for You (advice from the experts), Beauty Notes (things to jot down for reference), and Dear Mr. Alfred (questions you asked the author). The pictures and illustrations will show you how to achieve the effects you want in skincare, makeup, and color.

I want to assure you, this book will speak to all teenagers of color. I have seen your faces: the gentle blending of fair skins with bold features, brown skins freckled from the sun, hazel eyes peeking through ebony lashes, or profiles shaped decades and centuries ago by Native American, Asian, or African ancestors. Whether your skin color is chocolate or bronze, I want you to feel good about yourself, look good, stay healthy, and appreciate your beauty heritage as a member of a global community. I want you to take your rightfully earned place with the world's beautiful teenage girls and seek the eternal future. You will be a confident, stunning, beautiful woman!

I look forward to meeting you,
Mr. Alfred

CHAPTER 1

Beautiful Skin

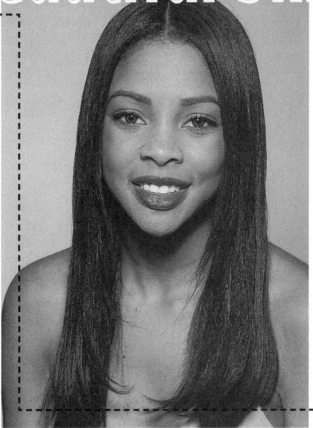

YOUR REMARKABLE SKIN can deal with almost anything. It adapts to stress, pain, and illness. It shrinks and stretches. It keeps out germs and bacteria—while it protects your vital organs and stores essential nutrients. It helps maintain your body temperature by preventing heat from escaping too rapidly. Your skin is your protector.

Your young, teenage skin is also sensitive. It works hard for you every day. So you need to understand it if you want to look stunning.

Skin Science 101

The part of your face that has the most stress to deal with is the layer of skin called the *epidermis.* This layer is what you touch, feel, and see when you look in the mirror. Actually, the epidermis is a series of layers, each slightly different from the one above or beneath it.

After washing your face and drying it with a facecloth, you may notice flaking skin on your forehead. This flaking process is constantly renewing your looks. The outermost epidermal layer falls away in pieces when it has absorbed all the stress and environmental impurities it can manage, and then the under layer takes its place. Until this happens,

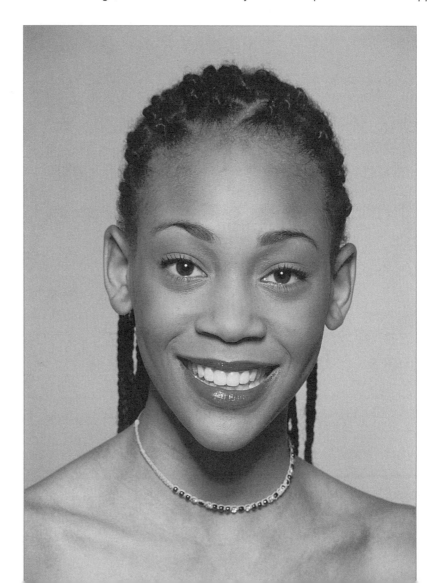

the under layer remains protected, waiting to supply your face with a new fighting army of cells.

Dark skin has more epidermal layers than white skin, and to some degree, this means greater protection from the sun. Dark skin often appears and feels smooth. It also reflects more of the sun's rays, giving greater protection and reducing the sun's drying effect. But for all these positive qualities, your skin needs plenty of help if it is to maintain its health and your good looks.

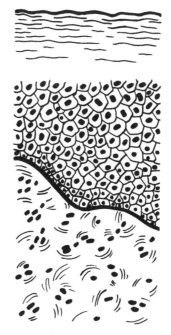

The upper layer of epithelial tissue, the under layer of germinating tissue, and the dermis, with regular blood cells.

Your Natural Protection

Two natural ingredients come to the rescue, helping your skin to do its job and maintain its "looks": water and sebaceous oils. You may have heard that oil and water don't mix, but in this instance these two elements work together beautifully to enhance and protect your looks.

Water keeps the epidermis moist, plump, and elastic, which is why you will hear so much later about drinking water. And oils act as a defensive shield and a reflector, holding the skin's surface moisture in.

If your skin ever gets too dry, oils alone cannot help restore its soft, youthful quality. Only water will do the job. If you soak a piece of dry skin in oil, for example, it will not soften, even if you use your own natural body oil. Remember: oil is not the softener; water is.

Sebaceous oils have another defensive purpose besides holding in the skin's moisture. They maintain what is called an acid mantle across the skin's surface, which helps ward off infection and skin disorders. Healthy skin is slightly acidic. Scientists call this the skin's pH factor. So when you see

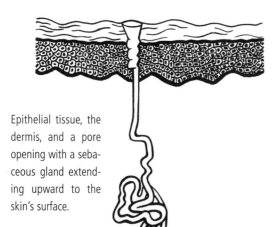

Epithelial tissue, the dermis, and a pore opening with a sebaceous gland extending upward to the skin's surface.

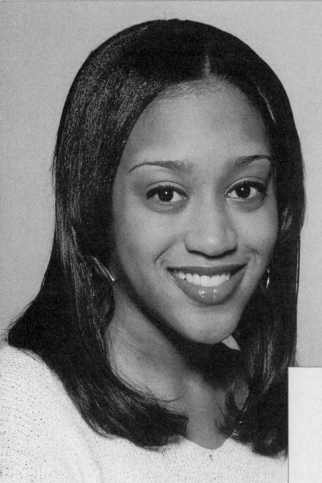

products that claim to affect the skin's pH factor, don't automatically accept or reject them, but just know that the skin's pH is important.

Your True Skin

Beneath the epidermis is the germinating layer. Actually, this is the deepest layer of the epidermis, which is also called the derma, or true skin. But the germinating layer is so different from the rest of the epidermis, that I think of it as if it were a distinct layer.

The germinating layer is maintained not by water or oils but by the blood circulated to this layer of cells. Whatever is in your bloodstream will show on your face, one way or another. Alcohol will show. Smoking will show. Drugs will show. A healthful or poor diet will show. Your skin is an indicator of your state of health. Moreover, your state of health will either help or prevent your skin from doing its job.

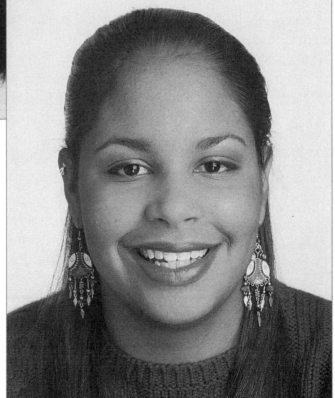

Now, let me sum up the don'ts and dos for healthier teenage skin. Remember: the effects of bad habits are very noticeable on skin of color, whereas the good habits are helpful to everyone. That's why I place the don'ts first. They can undo all the dos.

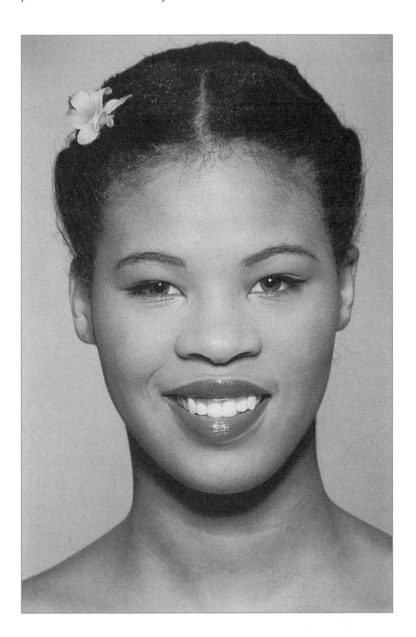

Watch Out!

Even though the outer layer of your skin receives a continuous supply of water from within, it may not be enough in all climates. Where you live affects whether or not your skin is in danger of going dry. Use a sunscreen or moisturizing guard to protect your skin from extremely dry conditions.

DON'TS and DOS
for Healthy Skin

Don'ts

1.   Don't consume caffeine.

Usually, the word *caffeine* makes you think of coffee and tea. However, for teens, sodas and some chocolate candy are the greater caffeine culprits. Caffeine increases stress, which can show up in your face. New studies have found that caffeine can make your kidneys and bladder work harder than they should.

2.   Don't overeat.

Being overweight affects the condition of your skin. The stored fat accumulates peroxides, which can leave the body more open to attacks, including allergies. The fat content of foods like chips, cookies, cakes, candy, and fries is not good for your health or your skin.

3.   Don't smoke.

Smoking cuts down on the amount of oxygen getting to the tissues, resulting in impaired circulation and a breakdown of good skin tissue. The results are dry lips, dry areas around the nose and eyes, and a dull, ashy complexion. Nicotine is a toxic substance—a poison. Planning to get married one day and have a healthy family? Your pediatrician and nutritionist will certainly advise you against smoking, as this nasty habit can put the health of your baby at risk. Ask yourself why you smoke. It's not healthy, chic, or cool!

4.   Don't drink alcohol.

Alcohol can rob your skin of vitamins and minerals—especially B_1, which is necessary for healthy skin. "Lite" just means a lower content of alcohol, but it's still alcohol. And remember that the "coolers" so popular in the spring and summer are alcoholic beverages, too.

5.   Don't stay in the sun for long periods.

Avoid sunburn. Because they are young, teenagers often feel that the sun will not harm them. But ultraviolet rays from the sun dry out the skin. The deeper the tan, the deeper the moisture loss. Dry skin loses its softness and suppleness, giving a dry, aged look. Without sufficient moisture, even creams can only do so much good. Later on in life, the skin will lose its flexibility and develop lines and wrinkles. It may take years to see the real damage, but once done, it is just about irreversible. I have taken care of the skin and applied colorful makeup to some very beautiful women the world over. I have met many young and maturing women, and the lines on their faces testify to how the sun has permanently damaged their skin. The skin feels and looks leathery, and the prominent lines around the eyes, cheek, and mouth area are not attractive. The word here is *caution.*

6.   Don't take too many long baths in the winter.

Long baths in the winter remove the protective oils from the skin, which are helping to keep the necessary skin moisture in the cells for suppleness. Once the oils are removed, moisture is drawn off. Even oil baths are not as effective as your natural oils—but do use oils, moisture sprays, and splashes after a bath.

7.   Don't use petroleum jelly and its by-products as a facial skin moisturizer.

Neither petroleum jelly nor its by-products, neither pure cocoa butter bars, sticks, nor its oil, should be used as a facial skin moisturizer. (If a moisturizer is water soluble, you *are* advised to use it.) Oils are not moisturizers and will not make your skin soft and supple. They will hold existing moisture in, but unfortunately the oils, if heavy or thick, can clog the pores, causing eruptions. Oils will definitely cause a shine, often giving a false impression of oily skin, when in fact, the skin may actually be dry. This is particularly true for those who are swarthy or dark-complexioned.

8.   Don't stay in or live in overheated rooms.

Overheated rooms usually are dry and will evaporate the moisture from your skin, causing it to become dry and flaky.

9. Don't leave makeup on overnight.

Always remove your makeup before going to bed. If left on too long, makeup can irritate your skin, clog pores, and cause eruptions.

Dos

1. Do exercise.

Proper exercise causes perspiration, which cleanses the pores and removes impurities from your system. It also increases blood flow to the surface, bringing needed nutrients to the skin. Try to get ten minutes of peak exercise a day.

2. Do drink eight glasses of water daily.

Your system needs water to function properly. Remember:

- Though water is something most of us take for granted, it is a cornerstone of good health.
- When you are dehydrated, water improves stamina immediately.
- Water makes up 75 percent of your body. If you don't drink water during an active day, then your thirst increases. This thirst indicates that you need water to flush your body with fluids, which will also keep your joints lubricated.
- Drinking water improves chronic indigestion by keeping food moving through your digestive tract.
- Water moisturizes the skin, cleanses the pores for a clear complexion, and flushes out poisons.
- Don't substitute soda, coffee, or beer for water. Medical experts advise that alcohol is absorbed into the skin and causes dehydration.
- New research studies confirm that water alleviates some asthma problems by loosening mucus in the lungs and curing the common cold.

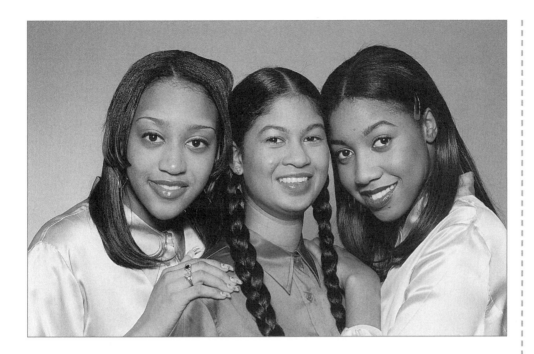

3. Do use a water filter.

Use a filter that draws off minerals and trace elements from your tap water. Using filters is cheaper in the long run than buying bottled water and provides you with water that is equally tasty. Your ice cube water should be as pure as your drinking water. If you buy bottled water, notice that:

Spring water usually comes from underground springs.

Mineral water contains calcium, magnesium, iron, sodium, and other minerals.

Sparkling water is carbonated and from an underground source.

Purified water has been distilled and filtered to remove minerals and any contaminants.

4. Do eat properly.

A vegetarian diet can contribute to healthy skin. If you are not a vegetarian, however, choose your diet with care. Eat raw, steamed vegetables, fish, and chicken. Limit your intake of red meat, candy, desserts, and sugar in general; tea and coffee; and sodas. Many young classical dancers and athletes take cod liver oil, zinc, vitamins C and E, and lecithin. Before you start taking these or other vitamin supplements, such as minerals and amino acids, consult your physician or dermatologist. If you are eating properly, you may not need them.

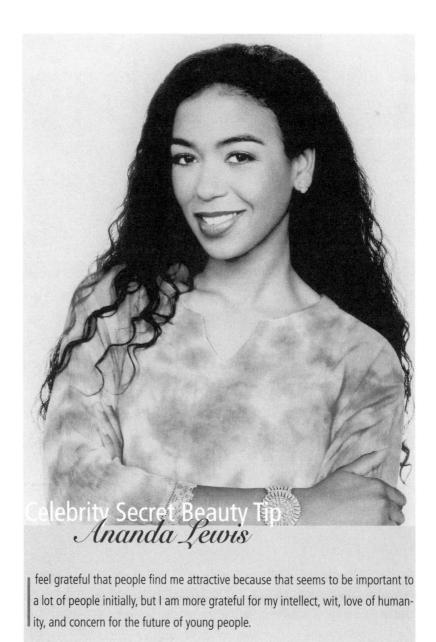

Celebrity Secret Beauty Tip

Ananda Lewis

I feel grateful that people find me attractive because that seems to be important to a lot of people initially, but I am more grateful for my intellect, wit, love of humanity, and concern for the future of young people.

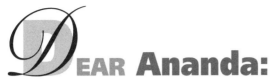

Dear Ananda:

How do you manage to always look so natural when you wear makeup?

—MELODY
Atlanta, Georgia, age 16

Dear Melody:

I drink a lot of water to keep my system flushed and my skin moist and fresh. My daily skincare product regimen is vital, and when I'm not on camera I usually wear earth-tone colors for a natural look.

—ANANDA LEWIS

What's the Sun Got to Do with It?

You may have heard that dark skin has more melanin than light skin. This abundance of dark pigment provides some protection from ultraviolet rays. But prolonged unprotected exposure to the sun can irritate even our dark skin. Unfortunately many black teenagers go sunbathing without applying any sunscreen. These long or consistent short periods in the sun can cause in teenagers premature lines to form between and around the eyes, toward the temple areas, and around the mouth. The skin becomes blotchy, and more uneven skin tones develop.

According to many dermatologists, sun protection—liquid sprays, gels, lotions, and creams—is often applied after the harm is done, when discomfort is experienced from "the slow burn," after the sun has gone down.

Many black teenagers that I've talked to who live in sunny climates tell me, "Our ancestors have survived the sun below the equator for centuries." Well, this is true.

However, our African sisters and brothers are no fools and use good common sense; and in their wisdom, they cover up the head as well as the entire body during the hot sun-filled workday. There is little movement during the midday, and most take advantage of the shaded areas.

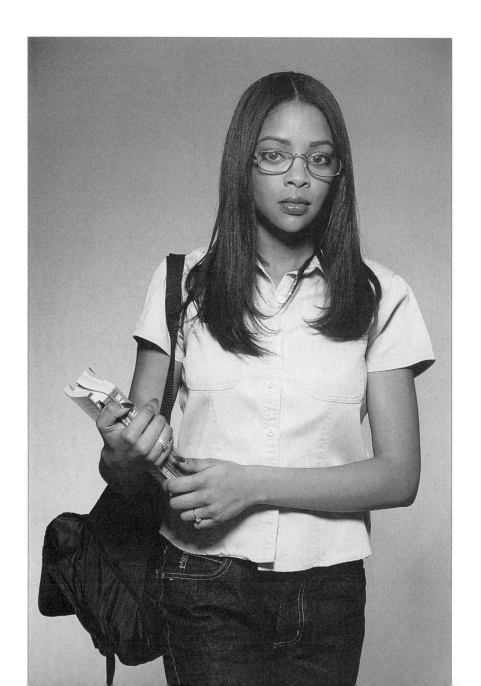

Sunscreen Protection

SPF (sun protection factor) is a rating index guide to help you make decisions in buying the appropriate sun product for long- and short-term exposures—for example, when skiing the snowy slopes of Vermont, in-line skating in the city, attending a golf or tennis clinic, horseback riding, playing volleyball, fishing, participating in a mean double Dutch jump rope competition with all of the girls on the block, and, of course, sunbathing and swimming.

Waterproof sunscreen formulations are excellent for all skin types. Here are the latest sun product formulations:

Forms of Sun Protection

- Liquid sprays
- Gel
- Lotion
- Cream

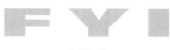

LIPS

Lips require full time maintenance: SPF 15–25. Your lips have no lubricating, oil-producing pores. The sun can burn and dry out the lip surface.

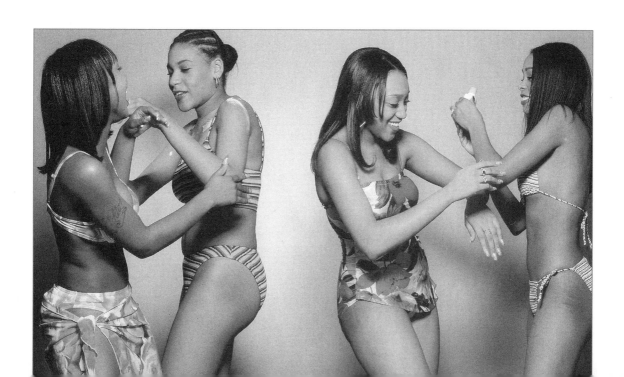

SPF Solar Index Guide		
Minimal protection		
4 to 5	Fast burn; great tan/least protection	Sunscreen
Moderate protection		
8 to 15	Slow burn; almost no tan	Sunscreen
Maximum protection		
15 to 30	Slow to no burn; optimal sunblock; takes longer to tan	Sunblock

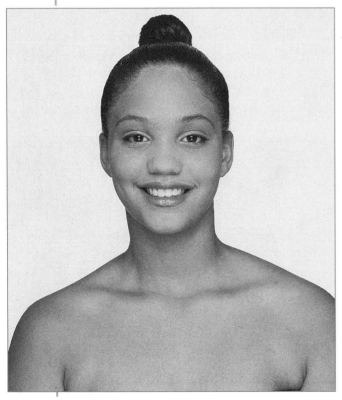

Your Skin Type

Do you think that your skin tends to be dry or that it tends to be oily? Perhaps it is a combination. Perhaps it changes from week to week. Your skin may become dryer or oilier, or may be more sensitive than usual, based on whether it is spring/summer or fall/winter. Some of you may find that your skin changes as a result of your menstrual period or your diet.

The amount of melanin and carotene in dark skin will often cause light to reflect off it, or appear to, rather than to be absorbed, as it is on lighter skin. If there is any perspiration on the nose or chin, the center of your face may appear shiny. This shiny quality gives the impression that the skin is oily, when actually it may not be. In fact, the skin could be dry.

So many teens tell me that they are confused about their skin type.

By just looking at your skin you can only guess what type it is. The trick is to know what to look for. Here's what to do:

How to Determine Your Skin Type

1 Wash your hands first. Also have a box of tissues in reach.

2 Make sure you have sufficient light, meaning that it approximates daylight, and be sure the light covers your entire face. No part of your face should be in shadows when you look in the mirror.

3 Notice your T-zone. This area comprises your forehead down the bridge of your nose, and from your nose to your chin. No matter what complexion you are, you may notice light reflecting off the T-zone as you look in the mirror. Look to the left and then to the right of the T-zone, and compare how your skin looks. See if there is a different amount of light reflected on the left and right sides of the T-zone, compared to the T-zone itself.

4 If the sides of your face and the T-zone are the same, touch first your forehead, then the tip of your nose and your chin. If there's perspiration, gently wipe it away with a tissue. If you still feel oil, then your skin is *oily.*

5 Note any areas that appear different—either patchy, rough, or discolored. Patchiness and roughness are often signs of *dry* or *sensitive* skin.

6 Your face could have some areas that are dry and others that are oily. This is *combination (normal)* skin.

Test your skin type twice a year: once during spring/summer and once during fall/winter. But don't do it at the very beginning or end of the season. Use common sense. If the change in season where you live is very abrupt, evaluate your face sooner; if the change is almost imperceptible, do it a little later.

The Skin-Type Questionnaire

Here is the best way to take any remaining guesswork and confusion out of typing your skin. Answer the following ten questions. Match your answers to the four skin types: oily, combination, dry, and sensitive. Whichever classification most of your answers fall into is your basic skin type.

Determine Your Skin Type

Question	Oily
1. Before and after cleansing, can you see oil?	Always
2. Does your skin feel greasy or slick?	T-zone; all over
3. If you bathe with deodorant soap, how do your face and body skin feel after an hour, without any type of moisturizer?	Oily foreheads, eyelids, nose, and chin
4. What do your pores look like?	Wide, enlarged all over
5. Do you have blackheads or whiteheads?	Many; summer problems
6. Do you break out?	Frequently
7. Do you peel or crack around the forehead, eyes, nose, mouth, lips, and chin?	Not in summer; occasionally in winter, especially around nose and mouth
8. Does your skin look tight, smooth, and ashen?	Rarely
9. Does your cleanser and moisturizer sit on top of your skin or disappear immediately into it?	Never disappears
10. How do you react to sun?	Rarely burn, good tan

TEEN TIP

My skin has always been about the same. But, sometimes when it gets dry, I just drink lots of water and moisturize my skin a lot.

—JAMILAH
Mt. Vernon, New York, age 14

Combination (Normal)	Dry	Sensitive
Sometimes; oily in spring/summer, dry in fall/winter	Rarely	Sometimes; summer problems
T-zone	T-zone; summer	T-zone; sometimes
Slightly dry looking in appearance and feel on jawline and around eyes in fall/winter	Taut, tight, and dry in feeling and appearance with ashen, dull cast	Tight and shiny T-zone after first half hour; sometimes in winter
Enlarged in T-zone, especially on nose, cheek, and chin	Almost invisible, fine pores	Noticeable in T-zone, fine elsewhere
T-zone problems; cheeks	Few; summer problems	Occasionally
Occasionally	Rarely; few in summer	Always; rashes and patches
Occasionally	Frequently; around eyes, forehead, mouth, lips, and chin, especially in winter	Occasionally; around eyes and nose
Sometimes; winter	Frequently; on forehead, cheeks, jawline, and chin	Rarely
Sometimes disappears	Always disappears immediately	Sometimes disappears
Slow burn, especially in summer	Burn easily without sun protection	Burn easily without sun protection

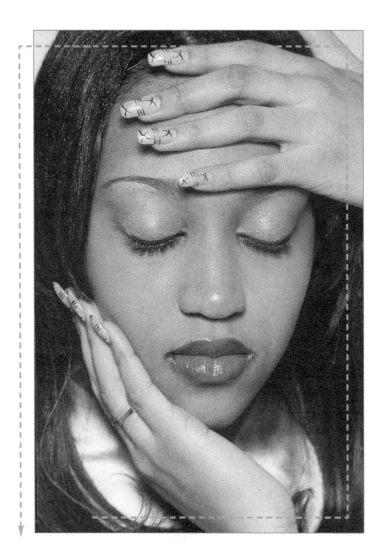

QUIZ WHAT DO YOU KNOW NOW ABOUT YOUR SKIN?

1 **Q.** Does your skin shrink or does it stretch?
  A. Both.

2 **Q.** What is the epidermis?
  A. The skin's outer layer.

Chapter Nine

Adding the Special Needs Trust to a Will or Living Trust

Should You Make a Will or Living Trust? 132
    Advantages of a Will 132
    Advantages of a Living Trust 133

If You Already Have a Will or Trust 134
    Modifying a Will 134
    Modifying a Revocable Living Trust 134

Adding a Special Needs Trust to a Revocable Living Trust 137
    Using *Quicken WillMaker Plus* 138
    Using *WillMaker*: Individual Trust 138
    Using *WillMaker*: Shared Trust 140
    Using *Make Your Own Living Trust*: Individual Trust 143
    Using *Make Your Own Living Trust*: Shared Trust 146

Adding a Special Needs Trust to a Will 150
    Using *Nolo's Simple Will Book* 151
    Using *Quicken WillMaker Plus* 152

Using a Will or Trust to Leave Property to a Pooled Trust 152
    If You Sign Up With a Pooled Trust Now 153
    If You Don't Sign Up Now 154

Sample Revocable Living Trust With Special Needs Trust 155

To make your special needs trust effective at your death, you must add it to a will or a revocable living trust. This chapter explains how to incorporate the special needs trust language (from Chapter 8) into your will or trust.

Should You Make a Will or Living Trust?

You can use either a will or a revocable living trust to put your special needs trust into effect. For most people, the better option is the trust, but depending on your family circumstances, a will may be the document of choice.

Advantages of a Will

In certain situations, a will is likely to serve you better than a revocable living trust.

If you are creating a special needs trust for a disabled spouse, you must use a will to keep SSI and Medicaid from counting the trust property as a resource. This is a special rule for interspousal transfers. It doesn't apply to other special needs trusts funded by a third party.

EXAMPLE: Harold and Maude are both 62 years old. Maude has multiple sclerosis and will need SSI and Medicaid if she outlives Harold. Harold wants to create a special needs trust for Maude, but has learned that the trust assets will be considered as a resource countable against Maude's SSI and Medicaid eligibility, unless he uses a will to create the special needs trust.

Cost. Wills are cheaper to prepare than revocable living trusts if you are hiring a lawyer, although the cost of including a special needs trust in the will is likely to increase the price. If you are creating the document yourself, there's really no cost advantage to a will.

Ease of change. Wills are easier to change as you go along. All you need to do is go back to the old document on your computer, make your changes, print out the new will, and sign it in front of witnesses. You can just tear up the old one. With a trust, however, amendments must be prepared, added to the original, and notarized.

No extra steps after you sign the document. You can leave property through your will just by listing it there. To pass it through your living trust, however, you must transfer title to the property into your name as trustee—for example,

3
Q. What is the skin's renewing process?
A. Shedding dead skin cells from the outer layer.

4
Q. What does air-conditioning do to your skin?
A. It draws moisture from it.

5
Q. What does water do for your skin better than oil?
A. Water softens your skin.

6
Q. If your pores are clogged, what might happen?
A. You could get acne.

7
Q. What do caffeine, alcohol, and smoking have in common?
A. They affect your health and the condition of your skin.

8
Q. When would your skin be in danger of going dry?
A. If the skin's loss of water to the atmosphere exceeds its upward supply.

9
Q. What are the four ways your skin could be classified?
A. Oily, dry, sensitive, and combination (normal).

10
Q. What do your lips lack that causes the sun to burn and dry out their surface?
A. Your lips have no lubricating, oil-producing pores.

Basic Beauty Facts

So many teenagers buy the wrong products for their faces, thinking that they have sensitive skin because their faces break out. This is money wasted and keeps a skin problem unresolved.

CHAPTER 2

The Basics of a Flawless Complexion

Love Your Skin

Now that you have determined your skin type, you're headed in the right direction.

Your next step toward healthy skincare and maintenance is cleansing your skin properly. Clean skin imparts a soft, smooth, comfortable glow and really feels good. So let's start now with a proper skincare program. First, here are some surprise tips:

Tips for Great Skin

- I don't recommend using soaps on your face, because most soap bars are highly alkaline, and usually the skin will become dry, irritated, patchy, blotchy, and discolored.

- Skip petroleum jelly. Many teens think of petroleum jelly as a facial "de-asher"; from the neck down, it becomes the all-purpose "ash-killer." Your skin may look like it's taking on a healthy sheen, but you're really doing more harm than good.

The basic steps to your quality skincare regimen are very simple:

1 cleanse

2 tone

3 moisturize

Then we'll add a special beauty step.

Cleanser Basics

- Match your cleanser to your skin type. When you go to the store, buy a cleanser labeled for your skin type. The cleanser will help remove dead skin and the impurities embedded in your pores. The product should clean deeply but gently.

- Match your cleanser to the season. During the summer, teens with oily and combination skin should think in terms of lightweight or light-textured products such as water-soluble lotions and gels. These clean gently and have less detergent, which produces less of a drying effect on the skin. In the winter, teens with dry skin might look to creams and rich emollients.

- When choosing a cleanser, make sure the ingredients are not harmful or abrasive to the skin. Some general cleaners contain grains, which remove the outer layer of skin. But

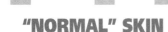

"NORMAL" SKIN

What you might call "perfect" skin, we in the cosmetics field call "normal" skin. Normal skin is facial tissue with few blemishes, and very little roughness or peeling. Many of you may have such skin. Normal skin has a uniform coloration that permits the upper skin layer to admit and reflect light (translucency), with unclogged pores.

when the grains are chips of shells or nuts, they often have pointed, sharp edges that can scrape, split, and damage the outer layer of facial skin. Natural grains, unlike shells and nuts, are rounded and will not cut or cause such damage; they dissolve as you gently massage and scrub.

- Try more than one product for your skin type, because each will be a little different. When you find the cleanser you like best, stay with it until you type your skin again, when there might be a need for a change, or if your skin reacts to the product.

- Remember, if your skin breaks out, it may not be the cleanser. First examine your diet or general health (see chapter 6). Then look to stress. Generally, your cleanser will not be the cause. Of all beauty products, skin cleansers are the most research and tested.

TEEN TIP

For a healthy complexion, you should just make sure you always use the right stuff on your skin. Test the product on a small spot before using it all over your face.

—GENNA
Montclair, New Jersey, age 14

Toner Basics

Products used for toning the skin are also called astringents, skin fresheners, refining lotions, and clarifying lotions.

- Choose a mild toner suited to your skin type. You will apply it with a cotton pad or ball.

- A toner rinses off any cleanser or soap film on the face. Its other purpose is to prepare your skin to receive a moisturizer. And it has yet another purpose. A toner restores the skin's pH to a proper level and corrects the balance of oil and water on the skin's surface.

- Your toner (astringent, freshener, or clarifying lotion) should be fragrance free, as well as irritant free.

- A toner is particularly important for those teens with oily, dry, or sensitive skin.

Moisturizer Basics

- Moisturizers do different things for different skin types. However, they will do the following for all skin types: become a sealer to hold skin moisture in (emollients) and draw moisture from the air to the skin to help keep it lubricated (humectant).

- If your skin is dry, choose a moisturizer to lubricate and protect your face with an oil-based mixture, which adds necessary oil.

- If your skin is oily, then your moisturizer should be oil free, for your skin has all the oil it needs. The moisturizer should also be water based, fragrance free, and dermatologically tested, since oily skin has a tendency to be sensitive.

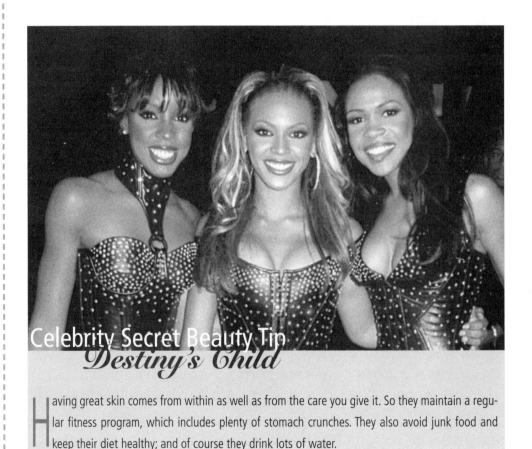

Celebrity Secret Beauty Tip

Destiny's Child

Having great skin comes from within as well as from the care you give it. So they maintain a regular fitness program, which includes plenty of stomach crunches. They also avoid junk food and keep their diet healthy; and of course they drink lots of water.

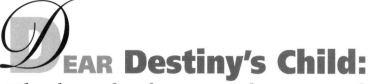

ᗪEAR **Destiny's Child:**

What do you do to keep your makeup so neat when you are performing?

—ALICIA
Phoenix, Arizona, age 13

Dear Alicia:

First of all, proper skincare first is very important. This keeps the oils properly balanced and after our makeup is on, we always finish it off with translucent powder.

—DESTINY'S CHILD

- If you have combination skin, then when choosing a moisturizer consider the time of the year and the overall condition of your skin.

- If it's winter and your skin is dry in places (for example, on your jaw or chin), use in those areas a moisturizer for dry skin and one for normal skin elsewhere.

- If it's summer and your T-zone is oily, choose a moisturizer for oily skin.

Eyes

The skin around your eyes is the most delicate, with the thinnest and fewest layers. When cleansing, use the mildest nonabrasive cleansers, and remember to use your fingers gently in this area and to move them from the temple toward the bridge of your nose.

All too often, teens apply mineral oil, petroleum jelly, or cocoa butter to the eye area. This suffocates the tissue around the eyes; because it cannot breathe it swells and gets puffy. This is exactly what you don't want. Always use a specially formulated eye oil—a lightweight, refined oil cream or gel for this delicate area. Massage the cream or gel in, gently patting it on with your ring finger, and working from the temple down to the nose.

For teens with oily skin, I recommend oil-free eye preparations to lubricate this area.

REVIEW

Every Morning and Evening for Skincare Success

1 Cleanse with cleansing cream, lotion, gel, or specially formulated facial soap.

2 Apply toner, astringent, or freshener, wiping gently with a cotton pad or ball.

3 Apply moisturizer with fingers or applicator. Dab the moisturizer on your nose, forehead, cheeks, and chin; then massage gently in upward and outward motions.

TEEN TIP

I would suggest that teenage girls test out facial cleansers to see which one works for their skin type.

—SYNCHANA
Harlem, New York, age 16

A Special Beauty Step—Facial Mask Cleansing

● Based on the time of the year and your skin type, I suggest that you indulge in weekly deep cleansing and treatment. By "deep cleansing" I mean to cleanse, tone, then exfoliate or mask with an exfoliating lotion, cream, or gel. These products reach deeper into the epidermis than can your daily cleanser.

● A gentle clay, lotion, cream, or gel mask is recommended for all types of teenage skin to keep pores clean and free of bacteria. Mask (exfoliate) once a week during the summer months and once a month during the winter. You might occasionally just need to spot mask (chin or cheeks only) if your pores tend to clog more often in these areas. When selecting your mask, always look for natural nonabrasive ingredients, such as aloe vera, apricot, oatmeal, sea kelp, cucumber, ginseng, and/or vitamin E. However, if you experience regular breakouts or skin eruptions, avoid using any over-the-counter masks until you've consulted with a dermatologist.

- When applying your mask, always keep the product away from the eye area. With the balls of your fingertips, apply with even strokes until the face is covered. Relax while your face is drying. (This ranges from ten to twenty minutes.) Rinse well with warm water. With the balls of your fingertips, massage gently, moving from the center of your face outward toward the hairline, and upward with long, gentle strokes from your chin area. Dry your face by patting, not rubbing with a clean white towel. Apply moisturizer. (The best time to do your facial is just before bedtime, so that your pores can close naturally while you sleep and you don't have to apply makeup or run around in the elements.)

Now that we have outlined the general skincare regimen, let's get specific.

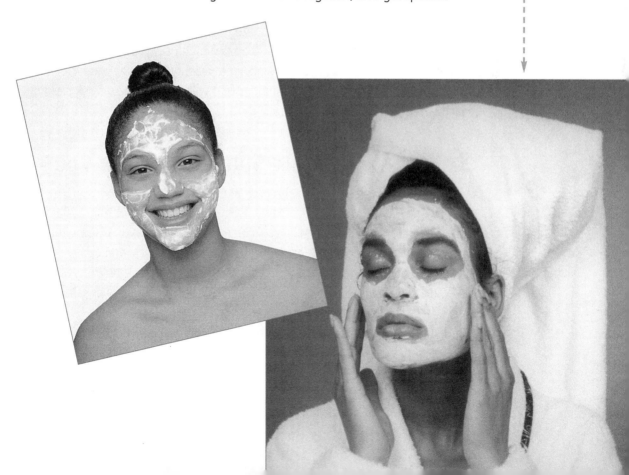

TEEN TIP

Exfoliation every once in a while is always good to brighten up your skin. Exercise always gives your skin a healthy glow.

—JAMILAH
Mt. Vernon, New York, age 15

FYI
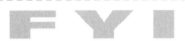

Facial cleansers are pH balanced and will not strip nature's protective acid mantle from your facial surface. Be aware, however, that some facial cleansers have exfoliation properties that include abrasive, mild particles that clean deep and slough away dead cells.

The Oily Skin Regimen

If your skin is normal to oily, this regimen will help you balance and control the oil. It's important that you drink eight glasses of water a day to flush your system of internal impurities and excess oil. Your oily skin systematically produces too much oil, day and night. If the sebaceous oil is not removed at least twice a day, your skin mantle collects oil, perspiration, bacteria, and impurities that will cause problems—for example, clogged pores, blackheads, and acne.

SMART *and* SENSIBLE SUGGESTIONS FOR YOU
All about Acne

According to Dr. Susan Taylor, "*Acne* is a very commonly occurring skin disease that is characterized by bumps, blackheads and whiteheads, large nodules, and cysts.

There are three primary causes of acne: clogging of the pores, overgrowths of a special bacteria that lives on the skin, or overproduction of oil by oil glands or sebaceous glands.

There are a variety of both over-the-counter as well as prescription treatments. The mainstay of therapy revolves around benzoyl peroxide products, which come in the form of cleansers, gels, and lotions, ranging in concentration from the low end of 2.5 percent to the high end of 10 percent. I recommend the lower concentration (2.5 percent)

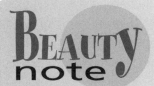

Acned oily skin is a medical problem and often requires the attention of a dermatologist. Ask a dermatologist about any acne products before you purchase them.

(unless your skin is very oily). Another common over-the-counter product is salicylic acid, which comes in a 2 percent concentration and is tolerated by most skin types. *My over-the-counter recommendation is the 2.5 percent benzyl peroxide applied at bedtime for six weeks.* However if there is any redness, irritation, or itching, please discontinue use.

Prescription acne medications consist of oral antibiotics and topical antibiotics, as well as retinoids. (Retinoids are a class of products that include Retin-A and Differin and Tazorac.) The retinoids unclog pores. Oral antibiotics include: tetracycline, minocycline, doxycycline, and erythromycin. Topically used antibiotics include clindamycin and sulfur compounds.

Oil gland activity, which produces excessive amounts of oil (or sebum), is one of the major causes of acne. An overgrowth of bacteria on the skin and clogging of follicles or pores also contribute to acne.

When we're under stress, hormonal levels increase and there's an increased production of oil by the skin, which in essence provides more food for the bacteria to grow. Pores are already clogged with dead skin cells, and hence we have acne. Dead skin cells and oil buildup absolutely contribute to the cause of acne."

People with oily, dry, and normal skin can be predisposed to acne. There is a hereditary component to acne. Acne can flare up if you are under stress or can be associated with hormonal changes before your period. Rubbing or scrubbing the skin can cause acne to worsen.

Acne can affect your self-esteem, particularly in teens of color. It's bad enough to deal with papules, blackheads, and bumps, but blacks have to deal with the dark marks that occur as a result of acne. These, in particular, can be a real source of emotional turmoil and upset. Try not to let it get you down. Go to work on it instead, like you're doing right now, by getting good information.

Susan Taylor, M.D.,

an exceptional physician who trained at the University of Pennsylvania and Harvard, is an internationally recognized expert in dermatology. She is board certified in both internal medicine and dermatology and lectures frequently both domestically and abroad. Dr. Taylor is director of the Skin of Color Center at St. Luke's Roosevelt Hospital and assistant clinical professor of dermatology at the College of Physicians and Surgeons, Columbia University.

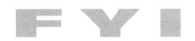

If you're out and about and find oil seeping and spreading all over your face, try a quick fix with "blotting papers."

Usually, oily skin has a noticeably uneven skin tone—light in the center of the face (T-zone), and slightly dark at the temples, outer cheeks, lower jawline, and chin. It is plagued with constant flare-ups and breakouts. Oily skin has visibly wide pores and a greasy, slick feeling. It can even appear dull.

A clean face is your goal. Oily skin must be washed at least once during the day and again before going to bed. (The ideal would be to cleanse your face at least three times a day, reapplying fresh makeup when convenient.)

Your oily skin is not an impossible problem when you know what to do. But you must plan your time and take care to meet your skin's requirements.

Day Care

Product to Use	Product Directions
Step 1. Cleanse Use lotion or gel cleansers that are oil and irritant free—they are less alkaline than soap. I do not recommend a cream cleanser on oily skin during the spring/summer months in any region. Use oil-free, water-based products researched for your skin.	Use tepid (lukewarm) water to rinse your skin.
Step 2. Tone Use a fragrance-free and irritant-free astringent formulated for oily skin. Skin fresheners and clarifying lotions formulated for oily skin are excellent for fall/winter.	Use lavishly. Apply with a cotton ball or pad and wipe until clean. Avoid the eye area. Also don't use an astringent that has resorcinol, a skin-darkening agent.
Step 3. Moisturize Light moisturizers are water-holding agents that protect, retain moisture, and shield against the environment. Use water-based, oil- and fragrance-free formulas for oily skin only. Oily skin types can have dry lips during all seasons. No oil-producing glands exist on the lips, so a mineral-oil lip moisturizer is excellent to protect your dry lips against the environment.	Place four dots of moisture lotion at the forehead, cheeks, and chin, and massage into skin. No residue or tacky feeling should exist. Apply a cocoa butter, camphor, beeswax, lanolin, or petrolatum lip moisturizer directly from the tube or pat on your lips. This formula is for lips only, and is not ever appropriate for the facial area!

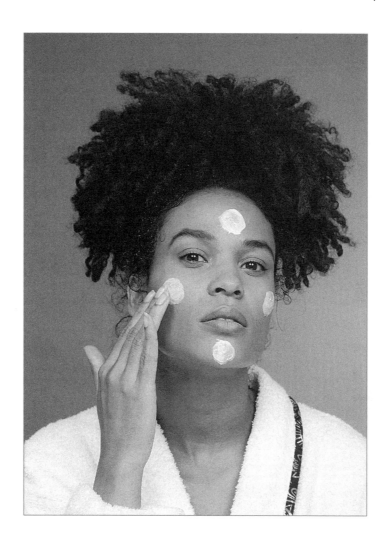

Evening Care

Product to Use	Product Directions
Step 1. Cleanse	Same as for day care.
Step 2. Tone	Same as for day care.
Step 3. Moisturize	Same as for day care.

Special Night Care

Product to Use

Use a water-based, oil-, and fragrance-free eye makeup remover. Use a formula for oily skin.

Product Directions

Use product with a cotton ball or cotton eye pad to remove eye makeup. Sweep gently with your ring finger from the outer corner of each eye toward the bridge of the nose. Rinse with tepid water to remove all traces.

Weekly Care

Product to Use

Use a deep-pore exfoliate or scrub formulated for oily skin. Deep-pore cleansing dislodges embedded dirt in the pores and removes the outer layer of skin-dulling dead cells.

Cleansing grains are great, but avoid formulas with sharp particles, as they can scratch and scar delicate skin tissue.

Clay masks with conditioning properties are best for oily skin, especially in spring and summer, if fragrance free.

Special Stuff

Have you heard of the triple-oxygen facial? Though quite expensive, it's for all skin types, but it is particularly good for acne-prone skin. The oxygen kills surface bacteria to help control breakouts and increases circulation for a healthy glow.

Maintenance Goal

Your goal is oil control. You don't want to deplete the skin's natural oil, but you do want to kill the shine.

DOS and DON'TS
for Teens with Oily Skin

Dos

1 Do drink eight glasses of water daily.

2 Do use only water-based, oil-free, and fragrance-free products.

3 Do use astringents as often as you can—day and night as well as weekly.

4 Do use a clay mask at least twice weekly during spring/summer, and once a week during fall/winter.

5 Do avoid fatty foods.

Don'ts

1 Don't use oil-based creams, lotions, or soaps.

2 Don't use acne-medicated cleansing pads as an astringent. You'll dry out areas around the eyes, temples, nose, and chin.

3 Don't use abrasive cleansing pads, buff puffs, or loofahs on your face.

4 Don't use *pure* alcohol, witch hazel, hydrogen peroxide, or concentrated lemon juice as an astringent.

My favorite scrubs are the ones with apricot and sea kelp. The facial exfoliating scrub gently cleanses away dull skin cells for a fresh-looking complexion.

The Dry Skin Regimen

If your skin is normal to dry, there is a basic regimen to help you maintain a balance between moisture and oil. It's important that you drink six to eight glasses of water a day to restore the body's moisture and to flush the impurities from your system. You should also know that dry skin requires serious attention.

Coating and pore-sealing oils—such as baby oil, mineral oil, and petroleum products—do not condition or relieve rough, patchy, flaking skin, and they sometimes can cause uncomfortably itchy skin. The ashen skin will disappear when these coating and sealing oils are applied, but they clog the pores and allow particles from the environment to stick to the skin.

Dry skin can look dull and gray or ashen, be sensitive, and often be painful. Its fine pores can clog and break out. The problem areas are the forehead, lower cheeks, jaw-

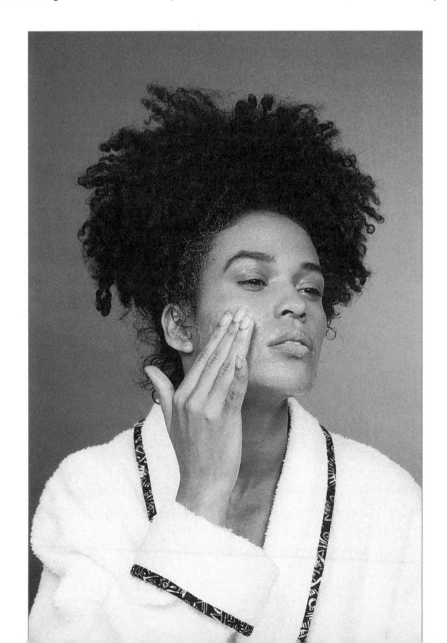

line, and chin. A dry, peeling nose can have fine dirt embedded as blackheads and whiteheads on the side and tip, invisible and unnoticeable, but sensitive to the touch. Dry skin reacts to extreme cold and hot temperatures, and suffers from a lack of both internal and surface moisture (dehydration), as well as from inadequate production of surface oil (sebum).

Day Care

Product to Use	Product Directions
Step 1. Cleanse Select a dry-skin emollient-based cleanser if your skin is extremely dry or a rich foaming formula if your skin is moderately dry. Also use rich emollients and conditioners and milk-based cleansing formulas designed for dry skin.	Tissue or rinse off. Massage gently, always moving upward and outward. Rinse with tepid water until your face is absolutely clean.
Step 2. Tone Use a nonalcohol toner for extremely dry skin or a low-alchohol toner for moderately dry skin.	Apply with a cotton ball or pad and wipe until all traces of surface impurities are gone.
Step 3. Moisturize Select a rich dry-skin emollient with moisturizers and conditioners specifically for dry skin. I prefer the fragrance-free, dermatologically tested formulas.	Gently smooth in the penetrating emollient from the base of your neck, massaging from the throat area upward to the hairline.

Evening Care

Product to Use	Product Directions
Step 1. Cleanse	Same as for day care.
Step 2. Tone	Same as for day care.
Step 3. Moisturize	Same as for day care.

Special Night Care

Product to Use

Use a no-tear, fragrance-free, dermatologically tested makeup remover.

Product Directions

Use a cotton ball or cotton pad to remove eye makeup. Rinse with tepid water to remove all traces.

Weekly Care

Product to Use

Use a moisturizing exfoliant to slough and peel off dry skin. Avoid clay or drawing formulas because they remove too much natural oil and and moisture.

Product Directions

Apply a thin film of moisturizer over extremely dry skin before applying a gel peel-off mask. Cream the mask with healing conditioners—for example, aloe vera.

Maintenance Goals

Your goal is to replenish and maintain the balance of water and oil on your delicate skin surface. You want to rid the skin of dulling dead facial cells and impurities.

You must take every preventive step to lubricate and hold moisture on your skin. Harsh winter and dry summer air robs your skin of its natural moisture and oil. You can retard the deepening of any lines in your face by using moisture-conditioning formulas that penetrate the layers of the epidermis.

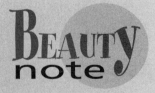

Your lips suffer in the winter. Use a mineral-oil lip preparation to trap and seal moisture on your lips. Medicated formulas relieve cracking, peeling, bleeding, and splitting.

DOS and DON'TS
for Teens with Dry Skin

------------------------------➤

Dos

1 Do drink eight glasses of water daily.

2 Do use only oil-based, moisture-conditioning, dermatologically tested products.

3 Do use a cream mask for very dry skin.

4 Do ventilate your daytime and evening rooms. Humidifiers are an excellent way to control moisture.

5 Do use spot facial masks during summer and winter, applying them to problem areas only.

Don'ts

1 Don't use astringents formulated for oily and combination skin.

2 Don't use abrasive, exfoliating, granular-based masks.

3 Don't use deodorant-type soaps on your face. From the neck down, deodorant soaps are fine.

4 Don't use petroleum jelly, cocoa butter, mineral oil, or baby oil as a facial moisturizer, especially if you are going to wear a cream or liquid cream makeup foundation. However, cocoa butter and petroleum by-products are excellent for the lower body parts.

The Combination (Normal) Skin Regimen

------------------------------➤

If your skin is oily, dry, or sensitive in different areas, then it requires special attention in both summer and winter. There is a basic regimen you should follow to maintain a balance between moisture and oil. It's important that you drink eight glasses of water a day to flush your system of internal impurities and to restore the balance of water and oil on the surface of the skin.

When in balance, combination skin can actually be normal. But seasonal conditions can affect combination skin to the point where it may be normal during one season but dry or oily during another. Additionally, stress, a dramatic weight loss or gain, dietary changes, and an irregular menstrual cycle can disturb the natural balance among acidity, moisture, oil, and dryness.

Skin eruptions, breakouts, and patchy rashes can sometimes occur on your forehead, cheeks, and chin. Your pores are fine around the hairline, temples, chin, and jawline but visible in the T-zone. Your skin can be part oily and part dry at the same time, so you must select appropriate treatment products for areas of your face and time of year.

Day Care

Product to Use	Product Directions
Step 1. Cleanse Use gel or foaming cleansers and oil-free and irritant-free cleansing lotions. There are water-based lotions and nondrying facial cleansing soap bars designed for normal to combination skin.	Rinse thoroughly with tepid water.
Step 2. Tone Use an irritant-free astringent for oily zones in summer. Use a skin freshener for normal to dry zones in winter.	Dampen a cotton ball or pad and wipe until ball or pad is absolutely clean.
Step 3. Moisturize Use a lotion or lightweight soufflé-type moisturizer. For lips in winter, use a moisturizer.	For summer oiliness, apply oil-free moisturizer all over, from neck to forehead. For winter dryness, apply soufflé-type moisturizer cream. Apply with fingers or applicator. Apply directly from tube or pat on.

Evening Care

Product to Use	Product Directions
Step 1. Cleanse	Same as for day care.
Step 2. Tone	Same as for day care.
Step 3 Moisturize	Same as for day care.

Special Night Care

Product to Use	Product Directions
Use eye makeup remover for combination-type skin.	Use product with a cotton ball or cotton pad to remove eye makeup. Rinse with tepid water to remove all traces.

Weekly Care

Product to Use	Product Directions
Problem areas: use a clay mask for oily areas. A creamy mask with soft grains helps draw out toxins and heals, firms, and alleviates whiteheads and blackheads.	Spot-mask the oily areas twice a month in the winter for 6 to 10 minutes. Avoid applying a clay mask to dry areas of the face.

Maintenance Goals

Your goals are to treat, care for, and maintain your normal-to-combination skin. Emphasis in the summer should be on the oily zones, and winter efforts are on healing and conditioning dry areas. Weekly deep-pore cleansing is important.

DOS and DON'TS
for Teens with Combination Skin

Dos

1 Do drink eight glasses of water daily.

2 Do use oil-free products that are light in texture for the summer season.

3 Do choose skin fresheners and toners formulated for normal and combination skin, based on the season.

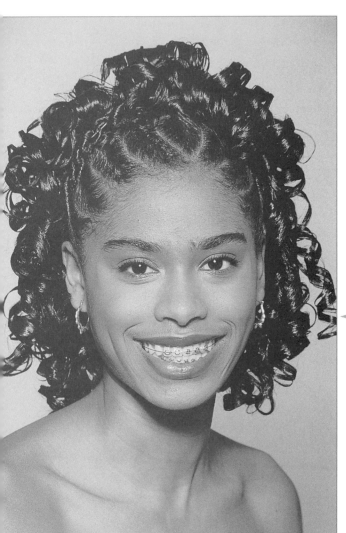

4 Do use products formulated and tested for normal and combination-type skin.

Don'ts

1 Don't use the same product year-round, because your skin type changes dramatically from season to season. Observe your skin and note the oily and dry areas.

2 Don't use abrasive cosmetic tools over the entire face, especially in the winter months.

The Sensitive Skin Regimen

If your skin is sensitive, there is a basic regimen that will calm, balance, and alleviate discomfort. It's important that you drink eight glasses of water daily to rid your body of impurities. Use fragrance-, irritant-, and oil-free products that are hypoallergenic or have been dermatologically tested.

Your skin type has less tolerance of chemical substances and reacts to poor dietary habits, stress, hormonal changes, allergies, trauma, impurities in the environment, exfoliating creams and lotions, and plastic surgery. It tends to be drier in certain areas and may have frequent skin eruptions. Your skin may bruise easily, resulting in dark spots. Cosmetics companies have made excellent efforts to meet the needs of your sensitive skin with products that are dermatologically tested to heal, soothe, and relieve your skin conditions and to improve your skin texture.

I recommend that you consult a dermatologist for treating extreme or severe sensitive skin conditions. And have a cosmetologist, an esthetician, or a beauty adviser do a patch test before you purchase a new product; you might even take a sample of that product to your dermatologist.

Day Care

Product to Use	Product Directions
Step 1. Cleanse In summer, use a gel or lotion formula. In winter, use a liquid cream or cream formula that is fragrance and oil free. Use products tested for black sensitive skin.	Massage gently with your fingertips. Rinse thoroughly. Tissue off or rinse off water-soluble creams.
Step 2. Tone Use a skin freshener designed for black sensitive skin, with low or no alcohol or resorcinal. Skin fresheners fight bacteria, balance the oil and moisture levels on your skin, and refine the pores.	Wipe the entire face, avoiding eye zones, until a cotton pad or ball is absolutely clean.
Step 3. Moisturize Use fragrance-free and oil-free lotions, or light, creamy soufflé-type moisturizers that are formulated for black sensitive skin. Fragrance- and oil-free moisturizers are water-holding agents that protect, condition, and smooth surface tissue.	In summer, your skin does not need a coating or sealing or moisturizer. In winter, apply a light film of cream.

Evening Care

Product to Use	Product Directions
Step 1. Cleanse	Same as for day care.
Step 2. Tone	Same as for day care.
Step 3. Moisturize	Same as for day care.

Special Night Care

Product to Use	Product Directions
Use a no-tear, fragrance-free, hypoallergenic, dermatologically tested eye makeup remover.	Use product with a cotton ball or cotton pad to remove eye makeup. Rinse with tepid water to remove all traces.

Weekly Care

Product to Use	Product Directions
Problem areas: use a clay mask to lift blackheads and draw out toxins and other impurities. Use peel-off or moisture-conditioning masks to clean deeply, lifting away accumulated dead cells.	In summer, spot-mask problem oily areas only. (This is not recommended for dry areas.) In winter, spot-mask on dry skin zones only.

Maintenance Goal

Your goal is to be as gentle as possible with your skin. Attend to breakouts or acne eruptions immediately. Your hands and fingertips carry microorganisms that breed on dirt, stale makeup, and polluted oil, so keep hands and fingers away from your face.

You must select a treatment system from one cosmetics company. Do not mix treatment products (for example, don't combine a cleanser from X, a toner from Y, and a moisturizer from Z). Fragrance- and oil-free water-based products that have been tested by dermatologists are recommended.

Now you know your skin type and have a regimen for daily care. Remember: take into account the season—spring/summer or fall/winter—when you answer the skin-typing questionnaire. And don't forget to ask yourself if there are any special changes going on: Are you dieting? Do you have your period? Been doing a "lot of partying"? Though I mentioned it earlier, it's worth repeating that your skin reflects your health and lifestyle. Since the germinating layer of your skin is fed through your blood system, what you eat and what gets into your blood system will have a noticeable effect on your complexion.

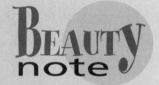

BEAU**T**y **note** Do not squeeze acne pimples, or dark scarring may occur. Do not use harsh cleansers or scrubs.

DOS and DON'TS

for Teens with Sensitive Skin

Dos

1 Do drink eight glasses of water daily.

2 Do use acne-cleansing pads without resorcinol, which is a darkening agent on black skin.

3 Do stay calm and learn to relax to help chase skin problems away.

4 Do develop better dietary habits. What you put in your body affects your skin.

5 Do use astringents or skin fresheners that have been specially formulated for sensitive skin.

6 Do keep your face's dry zones in check.

Don'ts

1 Don't use astringents designed for oily skin on the dry zones of your face.

2 Don't eat a lot of dairy products, salty and oily foods, or sugar-filled products, including chocolate.

Skin Problems

Pimples and blemishes, blackheads and whiteheads, moles, birthmarks, and discolorations can be problems. If you understand what causes these conditions and know how to cover or remove them effectively and safely, then you will feel better about your face and about yourself.

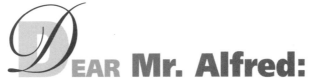 **EAR Mr. Alfred:**

The knuckles of my feet and hands are darker than my fingers and toes. How can I get rid of the discoloration?

—KIM
West Orange, New Jersey, age 15

Dear Kim:

First of all, check with your doctor to make sure that it is not caused by internal problems. Try giving your fingers and toes a weekly facial and exfoliate the dead skin away with a scrub. Use a bleaching cream with moisturizers on these problem areas daily.

—MR. ALFRED

Let's look at the skin "problems" most black teens ask me about. Remember, even if you avoid the "don'ts" and do the "dos" in this chapter, you may still have skin problems.

Breaking Out

There is no specific cause for "breaking out," but it can almost always be stopped or controlled. No matter what the cause, good, regular skincare can help. A healthy regimen plus internal medicine can cure most, if not all, incidents of breaking out and prevent their recurrence.

The type, form, and amount of medicine should be determined by a physician. Obviously, you don't need to go to the doctor for every blemish. But when you have a blemish that doesn't go away and it bothers you, seek medical advice. Yes, even acne is a condition worthy of a doctor's visit. Even if he or she is a licensed cosmetologist, the person at the cosmetics counter is a beauty adviser, not a physician.

Periods and Skin Eruptions

Yes, there is an established relationship between your periods and facial eruptions or breakouts. But preventive medication is available. Don't forget, though, that carefully cleansing your face before, during, and after your period definitely helps.

Blemishes

Blemishes are any skin faults—for example, blackheads, whiteheads, and pimples. When you see a blackhead, do not probe

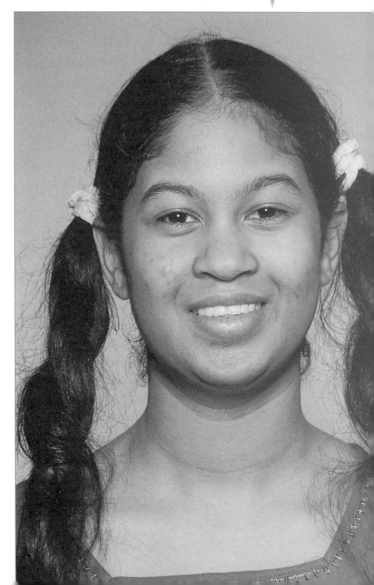

or squeeze it. Squeezing a blackhead can damage the surrounding tissue, and you can spread the infection to below the surface, causing other places on your face to erupt. The best way to remove or eliminate blackheads is to keep your skin clean. Remember, you can't have a blackhead without a clogged, oily pore. Therefore, the best approach is super cleanliness—morning and night, and sometimes in between.

The whitehead is so named because the head of the eruption is whitish in color. There are stubborn cases when whiteheads persist, and you should see a doctor or dermatologist, who will treat it with a miniature scalpel or electric needle. Whiteheads found around the eye (milia) are generally believed to be caused by abrasions or small cuts.

Blotches

To avoid blotches, avoid excessive sunlight. Limit the amount of ultraviolet light that hits your face by using a sunblock, either all over the face or on just the mottled area. Actually, *sunblock is a great base for makeup.*

If mottled, darkish spots already exist on your face, it is possible to have them removed through dermabrasion—the wearing down of the skin layers until the skin is clear. There are also abrasive scrubs and bleaching creams that help work off the dead, darkened skin. Ask a dermatologist which procedure is right for you.

SMART *and* SENSIBLE SUGGESTIONS FOR YOU
Mole Removal

According to Dr. Susan Taylor, "In terms of mole removal, they can be removed quite easily. Usually when they are removed, there is a discoloration that is left for a period of time. I do not recommend mole removal for teens (or adults) who have had keloids in the past. In terms of large scars, if they are keloids, and are raised, sometimes repeated injections of cortisone can soften and flatten them although not remove them completely."

Dr. Taylor continues, "Birthmarks can be concealed with makeup or can be treated with lasers and sometimes surgically removed, but some type of scar probably will remain."

Love Your Facial Skin Color

Now that you have a good skincare regimen to use every day, it's time for the "411" on achieving your most stunning look. Your skin color is the key.

Let's start at the beginning. Skin color is determined by three factors: carotene, melanin, and hemoglobin. Carotene gives a yellowish tinge to the skin, while melanin lends a brown color, and hemoglobin contributes a reddish hue to the skin. The more melanin, the darker the surface skin tone; carotene, on the other hand, provides contrast with a yellow undertone. The tone and undertone of your skin are based on the amount of carotene and melanin in the epidermis. For example, there are Africans from the Sudan who are so dark that they appear to have a bluish aura to their skin. This is directly related to the amount of epidermal melanin and hemoglobin in their skin.

All makeup is created to complement the undertone as well as the surface tone of your face. Teens today can change their hair color and can appear to have changed their eye color by wearing tinted contact lenses; but your natural beauty starts with your natural tone and undertone. The right foundation will help you enhance that beauty.

Foundation Basics

Many people think that foundation is primarily a concealer. But it's really used to impart a hint of color to your skin. Foundation is sometimes referred to as "base," "base color," or "makeup base."

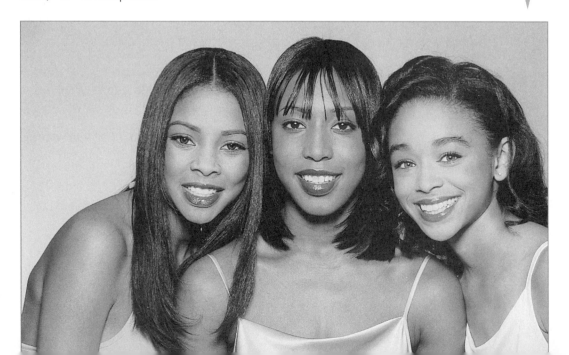

Uses for Foundation

When I talk to teens about foundation, I stress that foundation can be used to:

1 Protect against bacteria and impurities.

2 Even out the skin tones—that is, help adjust a light T-zone or dark, patchy areas.

3 Improve skin texture by providing a flawless, smooth finish; blushers and other makeup glide on easier and cling better when the skin is covered with a foundation.

4 Eliminate any sallow color (a greenish-yellowish or ashy cast), which occurs with certain skin pigment types.

5 Create a natural-looking healthy skin glow.

You should choose a foundation that perfectly complements your skin tone. To be able to choose properly, first there are some "don'ts" you should avoid.

What to Avoid in Choosing a Foundation

1 Don't try to change your skin tone with foundation. Sometimes, black models, actresses, entertainers, and opera stars have to change their skin tone to produce a certain stage effect. However, most teens appear in natural light or artificial light. It is important to choose a foundation that coordinates and harmonizes with your skin tone.

2 Don't buy a foundation without testing several colors in your skin-tone range. Test them in natural and artificial light.

3 Don't buy one foundation and expect it to impart the right color for all four seasons of the year.

4 Don't wear your friends' foundations. If a friend is in your color range, she might have yellow-olive undertones whereas you might have yellow-red. The foundation will therefore be different.

5 Don't rush when making your purchase. You can't rush into a store on the tail end of your lunch hour and quickly choose the foundation, especially if it's your first time or you have developed new color problems. You must take the time and have the patience to test your foundation, but first check your skin for changes and buy foundation accordingly.

Now that those don'ts are out of the way, here's what you should do. First, because your skin is dark, it is important that you test a foundation based on the season during which it is to be worn. As your skin gets darker or lighter, it can take on a golden-red, reddish-brown, or brownish-blue undertone, based on the amount of sun or wind it is exposed to. Don't look for an exact match; you are not involved in true skin-tone matching. For example, in the summer I suggest a summer foundation that cools down the yellow, red, and blue undertones.

Because you do not have a summer tan, your true skin tone can be better determined during the latter part of the fall and in the winter months. I suggest a winter foundation that imparts golden-beige, copper-brown, and rich red-brown radiance to African skin tones.

Bleaching Agents

You should also be aware that there are now fifteen cosmetics companies marketing skin-bleaching agents. These products permit you to even out your skin tone or fade out blotches and superficial spots. The bleaching product blends the shades of the spot and the surrounding skin. These creams also lighten the outer layer, giving an appearance of lighter skin. But when you use these bleaching creams, remember that your skin takes on a more yellowish undertone, since you have bleached out the dark part of the brown pigment in the melanin. This slight difference means you must rematch your foundation.

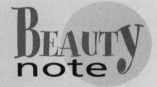

Plan a special outing with your friends. Make an appointment with a makeup artist or beauty adviser in a retail store or salon. Have the individual do a full-scale makeup application and take notes.

Your True Color

Your skin's undertone is the aura or glow of your true skin tone. It can be flushed out by standing in a room or in front of a white wall, with a white background, and in natural light. Wrap your hair with your whitest scarf or drape your neck and shoulders with a white sheet. Allow the ultraviolet light to bounce on your face until you can actually see a green (olive), yellow, reddish-yellow, reddish-brown, or blue aura.

For all their research, there is a skin tone that cosmetics companies find difficult to match. It is the tone in the medium range that has yellow or sallow, ruddy undertones. Black cosmetics companies and general market manufacturers have researched and developed foundations in literally hundreds of forms and shades. With some searching and patience, every skin tone can be matched to a color foundation.

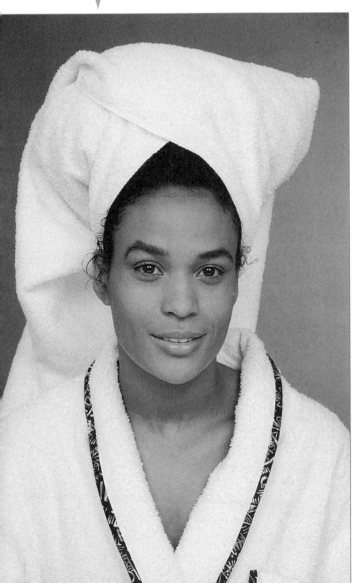

Your Skin Tone and Its Undertone

- Light skin. Fair—undertones yellow and olive; light skin—undertones yellow, red, and ruddy.
- Medium skin. Light or medium skin—undertones yellow-sallow; medium skin—undertones yellow to red and ruddy.
- Dark skin. Medium-dark skin—undertones golden, brown, and gray; deep, dark skin—undertones red, brown, and blue.

Types of Foundations

Skin Type	Formula	Coverage	Texture
Oily (use oil-free makeup)	Liquid/summer	Light	Matte
	Cream/winter	Medium/total	Semimatte
	Cream to powder/summer	Medium	Matte
Dry (use oil-based makeup)	Pancake cream	Total	Dewy
	Soufflé cream	Medium/total	Dewy
	Stick/tube	Total	Dewy
	Liquid	Sheer/medium	Semimatte
Combination (use water-based makeup)	Liquid	Sheer	Semimatte
	Cream to powder	Medium/total	Matte
	Pancake cream	Total	Dewy
Sensitive (use oil-free, fragrance-free, dermatologically tested makeup)	Liquid	Light	Moist
	Cream to powder	Medium	Matte

Create Your Specific Foundation Look

When you go to a cosmetics counter, especially one in an upscale department store, it is important to inform the beauty adviser or makeup artist of what you are looking for and what you expect from your foundation. For example, skin that looks oily and greasy is not attractive when foundation is applied. Likewise, dry skin can look dull, sallow, and ashen and will lack a healthy luster without a moist finish. If your skin is very oily and you prefer a finish with no shine or sheen, request a matte makeup finish. If you have normal-to-combination skin, you may desire an ultrasmooth semimatte finish (a slight shine). If your skin is dry, ask for a moist, dewy finish that will give your skin a natural velvet glow. There are some specific foundations that can give you a natural or soft velvet look. There are also foundations for problem skin that will still give you a soft natural look.

Create a Velvet Glow Look

Light to medium coverage is the foundation coverage for the teenager with an uneven skin tone, with blemishes, or with dull patchy areas and visible pores. When you use light to medium coverage, the skin takes on a very soft velvet texture.

Create a Smooth Refined Look

Heavier coverage is perfect for skin that has real problems: stretch marks, dark and light spots, superficial scars, dull sallow places, gray patchy areas, and blemishes. When applied properly, this foundation can produce an effect that appears very natural, without a masklike, heavy ashen look.

I do not recommend color washes, bronzing gels, or tints and color adjusters for black teens. *To date, not enough research has been done on black skin tones to convince me that these items benefit you.*

Blending Your Foundation

This is a very important step. When I say "blending," that is exactly what I mean: placing the color next to your skin and having it look natural. For example, many teens mistakenly apply foundation first to their chin. Instead, they should apply less foundation to the chin so that the color of the chin blends in more smoothly with the skin on the neck. You should always blend your foundation downward, using less and less foundation at the chin area. Always blend downward and blend lightly. The downward movement allows for better coverage without streaking because of the way facial hairs lie on the skin and hair.

If you are using a liquid foundation, place four dots of it on your face, then blend them together. (If you have oily skin and are using an oil-free product, be aware that you must use it rapidly because these products dry quickly—in approximately thirty seconds. If you are too slow, the dots will dry and you will be able to see where you placed them on your face.) The four-dot method is the best approach because you will not use too much foundation, and you will also develop a rapid way of getting complete and natural coverage on your face. One mistake many black teens make is to use too much foundation, believing this is the only way to get total coverage. Instead, put one dot on the forehead, one on each cheek, and one on the chin; maybe add one on the tip of the nose (this would be a fifth dot). Use your fingertips and blend the dots into one another, working out to the hairline and jawline.

The best tool for applying a soufflé, cream, or pancake cream foundation is a sponge. I am a firm believer in using a sponge. It is clean, frees the hands, and is better than your fingertips because the warmth of your fingers can cause streaking. But don't wipe your skin with the sponge. Use a press, dab, and pat movement. This allows you to place the proper amount of color where it's needed.

As you know, a sponge has holes, and as you press the sponge onto the surface of the foundation, it lifts away the product. So press quickly, lift quickly, and apply to the face. I don't recommend sponges for applying a liquid foundation, though, because they have a tendency to absorb too much liquid. Once you apply the liquid foundation with your fingertips, however, you can go back over your work with a damp sponge to smooth your foundation to the finish you want.

For those teens who use a soufflé with a liquid cream, a cream, or a pancake foundation, the sponge is the best tool for application. The cream stick is another item that can be applied to your face with a sponge.

The ideal sponge is triangular, so that it can be held between the index and middle finger and the thumb. Use a triangular sponge, employ the technique of press, dab, and pat. Don't wipe, scrub, or use a rubbing motion.

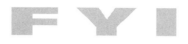

CREATE A SOFT VELVET LOOK

Light to medium coverage is adequate for the teenager with an uneven skin tone, with blemishes, or with dull patchy areas and visible pores. When you use the right foundation, your skin takes on a very soft velvet texture.

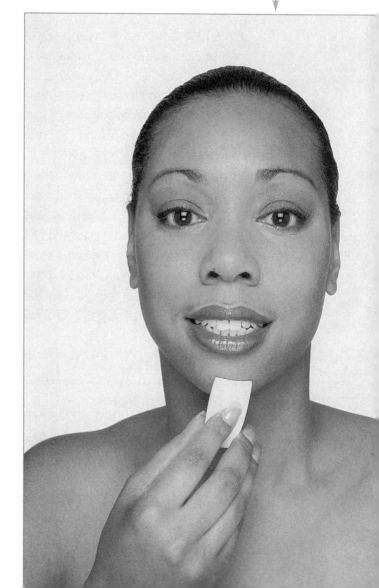

Placing the Foundation on Your Face

Where and how you place the foundation is very important. Once again, think in terms of facial zones. The center zone of your face is called the T-zone, which is where you should start to apply the foundation. Begin at the forehead and move toward the temples and around the eye area.

Circle around the eye area as if to get an owl-eye look. You don't want to put foundation on the eyelids or under the eye—just up to the rim of this area. The reason for using this owl-eye approach is that ingredients in some formulations might affect such sensitive areas.

If you have blemishes in these areas, use a cover stick or a concealer as a foundation for eye shadow and to erase any darkness under the eyes. Remember: your application movements should always be outward toward the hairline, but the stroking, pressing, dabbing, and patting motions should be lightly downward. This will encourage any

The Neck Area

Ordinarily, you should not have to put foundation on your neck. Your facial color, foundation, and neck color will blend unless you have severe discoloration.

facial hair to lie flat, since hair usually grows downward. Movement then is from the center of the T-zone, blending the forehead, temples, and under the eyes, then moving to the cheeks and then lightly from the cheekbone down toward the jawline.

You should lighten your application when reaching the jawline, so that your foundation blends evenly below the jaw. There should be no demarcation line between the jawline and the neck. You do not—and should not—carry the foundation beneath the chin and jawline onto the throat and neck. Application is from the center of your face outward toward the hairline. The movements are press, dab, and pat, stroking lightly downward to press the hair down.

Improving the Look of Your Skin

Some skin conditions that teens want to alter include blemishes, stretch marks, tattoos, birthmarks, and moles.

Remember that through good nutrition you can improve the health of your skin and thereby erase, retard, or stop some of these detractions. When this is not possible, or in the interim period during improvement, you can then use cosmetic coverings or concealers. But believe me, you can best improve the condition and look of your skin through diet.

It Gets Worse Before It Gets Better

If you have neglected your skin—particularly if you have oily skin with subliminal blemishes, blackheads, and whiteheads—your complexion may appear to get worse once you begin taking care of it. You may even find pimples you didn't see before. Don't worry. Your skin is a means by which your body rids itself of impurities. So when you cleanse and improve your system, you may well find your body expelling impurities through its facial pores, and this can result in temporary facial skin problems. Also, what you see on your face may be merely the blemishes becoming more visible as the dead outermost layer is removed. Thus, the blemishes are now closer to the surface and more visible—but also easier to address.

Concealers

If you are working to clear your skin, you'll see progress eventually, but you may want to use a concealer in the meantime. Let's discuss cover sticks (semiconcealers) and concealers themselves in the pages that follow.

Cover Sticks

A cover stick generally comes in a squeezable tube or lipstick-type tube. In either case, you apply the cream to the spot or area you wish to hide. The cover stick is generally used to help cover mild pigmentations and discolorations.

Cover sticks are excellent tools borrowed from the theater to conceal flaws anywhere on your face, with special consideration for shadows under the eyes, unwanted lines, birthmarks, scars, dark eyelids, and discolorations. Cover sticks usually come in beige-yellow tints in light, medium, and dark and are especially blended for you. If you have a medium-dark skin tone, use a cover stick a shade darker so as not to play up any lined and puffy tissue. The goal is to give the illusion that where the dark skin, upper lid, and area under the eyes come together is lighter, softer, and therefore smoother than it really is. In most cases, I prefer to apply the cover stick on top of foundation. The creams blend better and the cover stick formula stays put longer because it has something to cling to; also, it won't crease, slip around, or bleed. Use your ring finger to gently pat on the cover stick formula. On dry eyelids, use a cover stick to achieve a smoother finish to your eye shadow and to keep the shadow in place. You can also use a cover stick to contour your nose.

How to Apply a Concealer

If you are plagued with scars, pigment discolorations, stretch marks, and the like, concealers are good waterproof cover-ups for those large areas.

Most concealing cream shades blend easily with various products in their liquid, cream, and pancake cream foundations. For all skin types, these corrective creams are waterproof, nongreasy, and smudge free (a plus for oily skin). They easily conceal most skin imperfections, such as scars, burn marks, blotches, blemishes, circles under the eyes, birthmarks, stretch marks, surgical discolorations, and tattoos.

To apply a concealer for maximum effect, your skin first has to be "squeaky clean." The manufacturers supply directions for their products, but they all say basically the same thing: clean skin is a must before application. Then apply concealer directly to the affected area, using a spatula that generally comes with the product. Apply the product a little at a time.

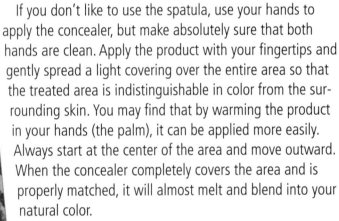

If you don't like to use the spatula, use your hands to apply the concealer, but make absolutely sure that both hands are clean. Apply the product with your fingertips and gently spread a light covering over the entire area so that the treated area is indistinguishable in color from the surrounding skin. You may find that by warming the product in your hands (the palm), it can be applied more easily. Always start at the center of the area and move outward. When the concealer completely covers the area and is properly matched, it will almost melt and blend into your natural color.

While the concealer is still damp, immediately apply the specially formulated powder with a powder puff or brush in order to set, seal, and dry the concealer. All of this must be done before you can touch the area. It shouldn't take more than a minute to apply the concealer and powder. As long as the concealer is applied rapidly and is still damp when you begin with the powder, you are safe.

Now you can decide whether you wish to use a foundation. Many of you will. Apply your foundation along the outer edge of the concealed area. Blend it in there and over the rest of your face.

The key to the successful use of a concealer is to pair the right concealer and foundation with your skin color. Then you can blend at the edges, or demarcation line, to achieve a flawless look. If the concealer and foundation match your natural skin color, you will have no problem following the directions and getting the required results.

Face Powders

Many black teens have decided that they do not need or cannot use powder, largely because they have gotten poor results. However, powder can eliminate the shine for you if your skin tends to be slightly oily.

Applying powder to your foundation also prepares your face, giving it a silky texture on top of which to apply your blush. However, some makeup artists want you to apply foundation first, other colors next, and powder last, to set the face.

Which method you use depends on your skin type. For this decision, I divide black teens into two skin types: those with oily skin should apply powder immediately after the foundation; those with dry skin should apply the foundation first, then the eye and cheek color, and set the face with translucent powder.

Types of Powder

There are two types of powder: translucent setting powders and shaded, or pigmented, powders. They each have different purposes beyond that of setting your foundation. Translucent powders are usually loose formulas, with a tint of either amber or bronze. These are usually termed translucent because you can see through the powder to your skin, which will have a glow. These setting powders are used to absorb surface oil and perspiration—for example, for touch-ups before work, after lunch, on the T-zone, and on the cheeks.

Shaded powders are for those who prefer to use a moisturizer and may not use a liquid, cream, or pancake cream foundation. They may be bought either loose or solid in a compact. Shaded powder is a pigmented powder that is applied over your moisturizer.

I have no problem with teens using shaded powders in place of foundation and translucent powder. Remember, though, that pigmented powder not keyed to your foundation coloring can disturb it. For instance, if you have a bronze foundation and you put a sable powder over it, the result will be a muddy look, giving the skin a gray, dull appearance. In contrast, translucent powders need not match your color skin. They are designed to set the foundation and absorb the perspiration and oil deposits associated with the foundation.

You do not have to worry about powders lending an ashy or gray look to your skin. If the color of your powder is keyed properly to your skin, this will not happen. It is titanium dioxide, a white talcum powder, which usually gives that look to black skin. Just make sure the powder you choose is the right color for you. In summary, some people want to have moist-looking skin while others want a semimatte or matte appearance. Powder should be used for the purposes suggested. If you don't want a shine, use powder. The option is yours.

The Benefits of Powder

I have already presented some of the benefits of powder, but now I would like to mention these additional ones, so that you will know what kind of powder to buy, and what to avoid.

The Pluses of Powder

1 Sets makeup foundation.

2 Absorbs oil and perspiration.

3 Does away with the shine.

4 Blushers glide on more easily and set better.

It is important that you use only translucent powder after applying foundation. You don't want to use *shaded* powders to dust or set your foundation. Because they can

BEAUTY MYTH

In addition, today's powders will not dry your skin. Many black women feel that powder causes a gray or ashy look. This is not true. Most powders have some type of moisturizing agent, and the amount depends on the brand. When properly applied, powders will impart a natural, translucent sheen to the face.

change the color, shaded powders are only good if you don't apply foundation. Also, remember that a little powder goes a long way. You don't need to use a lot of powder to set your foundation. A "cakey" effect is not attractive, and it emphasizes any lines you have under you eyes, around the nose and mouth, and even the cleft of the chin. Think of putting a sheer veil over your face; that is the amount of powder to apply. The ideal is to use powder to set the foundation and to allow the skin and color foundation to glow.

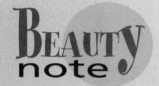 To keep your blusher on longer, try a light application of translucent powder over it and under it.

How to Apply Powder

Loose powder comes in a container with a scoop-out feature, so it can be reused without spoiling the entire product. A shaker container is ideal. It is like a salt or pepper shaker, whereby you can measure the amount of powder and control its spillage. There is also a compact powder. In this instance, you cannot shake or pour the powder, but rather, you use a flat puff applicator to lift the powder from the container to your face.

A cotton ball is usually used to apply loose or pressed powder. A powder puff is usually flat and is used for applying pressed powder. A fluffy powder puff is usually used for loose powder, while the fluffy powder brush, which is an ideal applicator, is recommended highly for loose or pressed powder application.

How to Get the Look You Want

What look do you want? The matte look is achieved with loose powder and the fluffy puff. Press, dab, and pat is again the operation in applying loose powder. To achieve a sheen (a moist look), again use loose powder, but apply it with a powder brush. To achieve an oil-free, perspiration-free look, teens with oily skin, or teens who do not want a shine in the T-zone, use pressed powder with a flat puff or a cotton ball. Pressed powder, in general, is ideal for oil absorption.

Some Powder Tricks

Use a loose powder whenever you want to soften a line of demarcation. These are usually under the eyes, along the hairline, and on the jawline. Loose powder is excellent for blending your undereye concealer with your blusher. Setting powder can easily be powdered between these two lines to soften the effect, or even erase it, resulting in a very natural meeting of color. The trick is to dip the powder brush in the powder and flick away the excess powder, then redip the brush in the loose powder and flip away the loose powder, and then dip the brush into the blusher and shake off the excess. Now you have both the blusher color and the loose powder on the bristles. All you have to do is fan the brush over the line of the demarcation to get a softened effect.

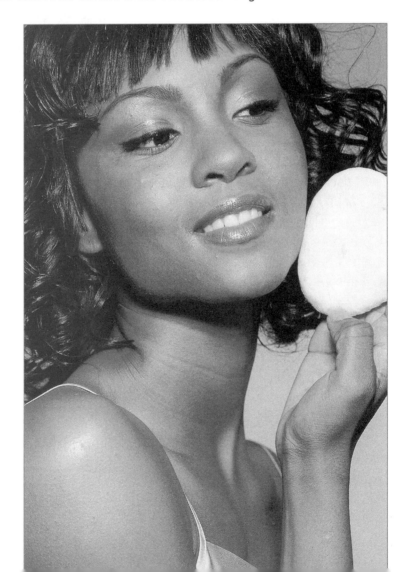

QUIZ   ESSENTIALS ABOUT YOUR SKIN

1   **Q.** How many ways could your skin be classified?
        A. Four ways—oily, dry, sensitive, and combination/normal.

2   **Q.** What is the primary reason to use foundation?
        A. To even out your skin tone.

3   **Q.** What are the three most important steps to your daily regimen?
        A. Cleanse, tone, and moisturize.

4   **Q.** What does translucent powder do?
        A. Sets your makeup and gives you a matte finish.

5   **Q.** What is the best way to tone down blemishes or dark marks?
        A. Apply concealer after you moisturize your skin.

6   **Q.** What should I drink to help keep my skin clear?
        A. Eight glasses of water a day.

CHAPTER 3

The Color Workshop

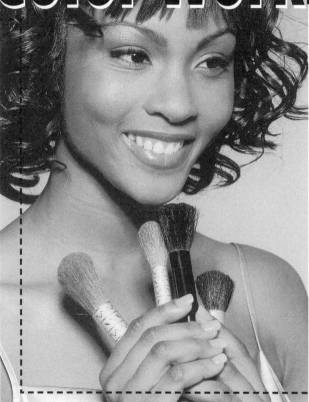

Choosing the Right
Colors for Your Best Look

Teenage girls of color come in many different shades, from alabaster to velvet-smooth ebony—some thirty-nine skin-color types! African American teenagers represent the richest spectrum of color found anywhere in the United States. You have developed a talent for wearing color with such incredible flair. So keep that fresh and open mind. Join me in breaking through the rules to enhance your beauty.

Breaking through the Rules

The adult beauty and fashion industries have taught your mothers, aunts, and cousins to believe that there are rules in beauty fashion that cannot be broken. Some will make you laugh and some may make you grit your teeth. I'm sure you've heard them all. Here's a test to see if you are ready to break the rules of beauty and fashion. Answer yes or no after each statement.

1   Bright colors are not for dark skin. _____

2   Brown colors should be avoided. They're too close to our skin color. _____

3   Bright pinks, reds, and yellows are for "loose" and immigrant women. _____

4   Blond hair is only for the bluest eyes. _____

5   Hair color is only for old ladies. _____

6   Yellow should be avoided by light-skinned blacks. It makes them sallow. _____

7   Black is for funerals and mourning. _____

8   White is a color everyone can wear. _____

9   "Big" full lips should be painted in muted soft colors, not red colors. _____

10   Paint your toenails if you must. Painted fingernails are for fast girls. _____

Your Undertones

Step One

Pull your hair away from your face and wrap a white cloth around your face. It will reflect the natural light and show your undertones.

Step Two

Stand with your back to a north-facing window and hold a mirror in front of you. A north window provides natural light, which is the best light for finding your undertones.

Step Three

Study your face. Take a good look! Examine your skin. Turn your head slowly from side to side to side. You will begin to see your undertones.

- Are they reddish?
- Are they yellow?
- Are they yellow-olive?
- Or are they blue?

Step Four

Look at your eyes. Look into the pupils. Some of you will be surprised to see that your inky black eyes are encircled in an inky blue. Or that those dark brown eyes have hazel or reddish flecks. Or that you have a light hazel right eye and a left eye with flecks of green, blue, or both!

Stey by Step: Finding Your True Colors

It's easy. All you need is:

- A white cloth, pillowcase, or towel
- A hand mirror
- Natural light
- Clean face devoid of makeup
- Ten minutes

COLORS TO AVOID

If your natural skin coloring is in light, medium, or dark hues and it is ruddy or sallow, then beware. Intense shades tend to drain color from your face. Also a note of caution about weak shades such as beige, heather, light mauve, and soft yellows. They can be terribly unkind to your complexion. If your skin is blemished, with spots on the cheeks or close to the earlobe, dark circles beneath your eyes or lines in your face, avoid violet and purplish grays. These shades repeat the colors of natural lines and shadows and emphasize them all the more. Having healthy skin obviously is the key to wearing color. If your skin is clear and has no unattractive tints, then almost any color can be worn.

Step Five

Examine your hair. Fluff it so the natural color can be easily seen. Turn your head from side to side and look for your hair's undertones. Your description of black hair now is changed to dark brown with reddish highlights, or dark brown with copper highlights. (Consult chapter 5 for more about hair.)

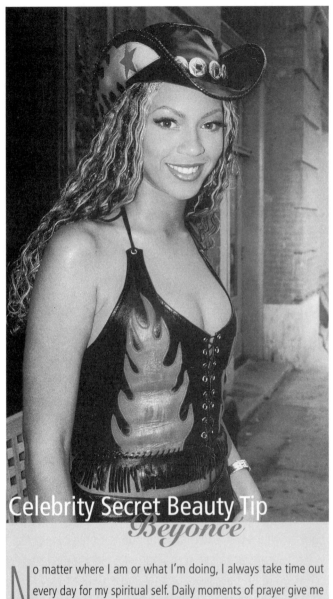

Celebrity Secret Beauty Tip

Beyoncé

No matter where I am or what I'm doing, I always take time out every day for my spiritual self. Daily moments of prayer give me my inner peace.

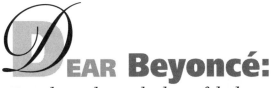

*D*EAR **Beyoncé:**

Your hair always looks so fabulous. What convinced you that blonde was the best color for you?

—MELANIE
New Haven, Connecticut, age 17

Dear Melanie:

I wanted a change, so I sought expert advice from my hairstylist, who did a few strand tests. We selected the best color to bring out my complexion.

—BEYONCÉ

The Flair for Color

Teenagers of color are born to wear unusual colors in every hue: Royal Purple, Mysterious Black, Exciting Red, Romantic Pink, Peach and Lavender and Earthy Coppers, Red-Orange, Terra-Cotta, Orange, Tan, Brown, and Gold.

Now let's learn how to combine colors and select shades that will make the most of your facial beauty—your eyes, skin, and hair. No need to take out a loan from your parents and spend all of your disposable money on makeup and hair. Color is what's happening. Black teens are setting the style.

Teenagers of color are on the move. Your presence and your beauty have left a mark in women's sports, music, modern and classical dance, religion, acting, fashion and education and will continue to do so as you continue to daringly break the color rules. So keep up the good work!

A New Eye on Color

Try black with white, green with yellow, brown with white. Yes, these color combinations work well and complement each other. But how about kelly green and shocking pink?

Or black and brown? Or pink and orange? The teenage girl who has dared to mix non-traditional colors that also complement her skin color has developed an educated eye. She instinctively sees the nuances in a shade of color. That blue is no longer just that—but is a teal blue with tones of green, periwinkle, violet, sky blue, or turquoise. So let's begin to examine colors more closely, so that you can select the precise shade that is most becoming to your skin.

QUIZ

1

Q. Which skin tone and eye color are most flattered by the color hunter green?

A. Dark brown skin with dark brown eyes.

2

Q. What color would be great for someone with both hazel eyes and light skin?

A. Coral.

3

Q. You have a medium-brown complexion and blue eyes. What are your best colors?

A. Gray, blue, and blue-green.

*D*EAR Mr. Alfred:

I'm sixteen years old and medium complexioned, with dark brown eyes. My favorite makeup colors are brown, green, and light blue. Please tell me what color lipstick would be good for me.

—AMILCAR
Harlem, New York, age 16

COLOR YOUR WAY

Matching Colors with Your Skin Type

Dark Skin:

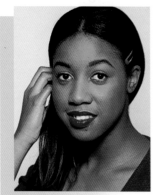

Dark complexions with grayed and red undertones look best with primary hues of red, mauve, and magenta.

Suggested Colors:

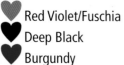
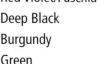

Red Violet/Fuschia
Deep Black
Burgundy
Green

Lavender
Blue/Blue Violet
Tan
Hunter Green

Complementary accent colors are: Yellow-Orange, Deep Gold, Black, and Chartreuse.

Medium Skin:

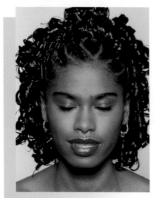

Medium brown and dark complexions usually look best in shades that have a bit of red added to them. In general, they are flattered by colors with blue, rather than yellow, undertones.

Suggested Colors:

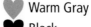

Pink
Lavender
Royal Blue
Warm Gray
Black

Blue-Green
Peach
Blue Violet
Gray

Complementary accent colors are: Brilliant Red, Teal, Orange, Tonal Blacks with neutral characteristics such as Gray or Black.

Light skin:

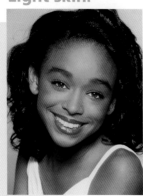

A teenager with fair, light skin with yellow or olive coloring will usually look best in shades that have an earthy yellow cast.

Suggested Colors:

Coral
Vivid Orange Red
Yellow-Green
Pastel Cream
Eggshell Yellow

Complementary accent colors are: Violet, Brown, Terra-Cotta, Amber, and Greenish Blue.

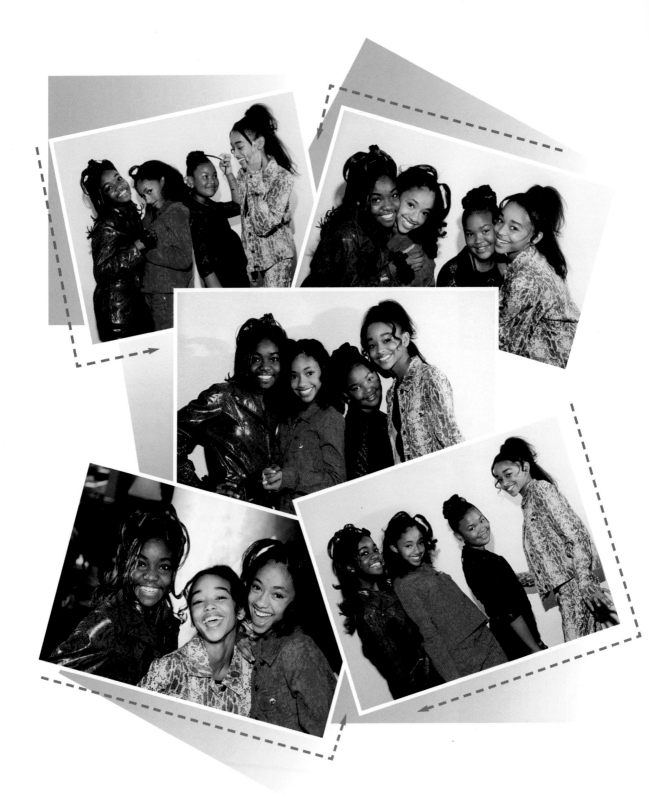

In the Eyes of the Beholder

The color of your eyes and their hues are illuminated if you wear a shade that matches or is slightly darker than your eye coloring. If you have light brown hazel, blue green, or green eyes, experiment with wearing a softer shade of eye color near the bridge of the nose and a more intense shade farther away to contour the eyes.

The Best Colors for Dark Brown Eyes:

- Blue-Black
- Black Gold
- Mocha
- Saffron
- Deep burgundy

- Black
- Vermilion
- Gold
- Frosted Tan
- Black Plum

- Silver
- Forest Green
- Cinnamon Spice
- Hunter Green
- Cinnamon

The Best Colors for Brown Eyes:

- Terra-cotta
- Shades of Amber
- Brown
- Navy Currant

- Sand
- Copper
- Green

- Dark Beige
- Gold
- Blue

The Best Colors for Hazel Eyes:

- Brown
- Coral

- Green
- Yellow-Red

- Blue
- Gold

The Best Colors for Green Eyes:

- Dark Shades of Green
- Shades of Gray

- Searing Brown
- Red

- Blue-Green
- Yellow-Red

The Best Colors for Blue Eyes:

- Gray hues

- Blue

- Greenish Blue

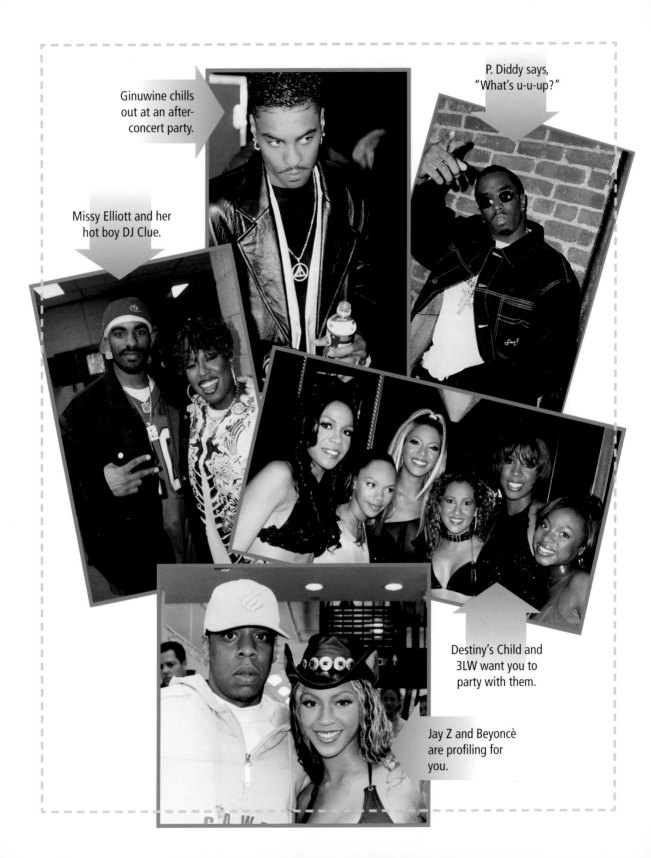

Ginuwine chills out at an after-concert party.

P. Diddy says, "What's u-u-up?"

Missy Elliott and her hot boy DJ Clue.

Destiny's Child and 3LW want you to party with them.

Jay Z and Beyoncè are profiling for you.

Dear Amilcar:

You're on the right track with your color choices. (Review my color chart for the full spectrum.) Blue, however, is your most highly recommended—royal blue, blue-black, blue-violet, and blue-green. And you would wear orange, cinnamon, pink, and red lipstick very well. Be daring!

—MR. ALFRED

Gorgeous Makeup from Day to Date

Now that you have determined what your best colors are, let's do accents! Your eyes! Your cheeks! Your lips! But in order to color your face, you need the proper tools. So let's see what they are!

Special Stuff

Try a little pearlescent eye shadow on the tips of your lashes for a fabulous flutter.

Your Color Tools

- Contour brush
- Powder brush
- Eyelash curler
- Eyeliner brush (optional, use if your lashes are very straight)
- Eye shadow sponge
- Eye shadow brush
- Brow brush
- Lash comb (optional, if you have extremely curly lashes)
- Lip liner pencil

● Lipstick brush

● Contour brush

Having these face-coloring tools is important, but you also must know the proper techniques and procedures for using them. Your makeup steps now come into full use. In the previous chapters we discussed skincare, foundations, and powders. Let's review the steps:

Steps for Skincare

1 Cleanse.

2 Tone.

3 Moisturize.

4 Apply concealer (optional).

5 Apply foundation, or base.

6 Apply concealer (optional for oily skin types). In my opinion, eye concealers, for example, perform better on top of the foundation and powder than underneath them.

7 Contour the cheeks (optional).

8 Apply powder.

Now you're ready to take that regimen to another level. Let's go on ahead.

We'll start with the application of eye makeup. Next, we'll apply blusher and then lipstick. You might prefer a different order, such as: blusher, then do the eyes, and then do the lips. You'll get the same fabulous results. The choice is yours.

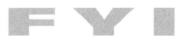

Eye shadow comes in dozens of colors, including pearlescent, matte, crème, and satin textures. For a special night out, touch a little to your cheeks to create face-flattering accents.

Your Eyes and the Use of Color

When I think of eyes, I think of Ananda Lewis, Beyoncé, Brandy—all with eyes that allure, hold, capture, and hypnotize you.

These are the faces of visible African American young women, and their eyes are made up to hold our attention. Because of this, many black teens tend to admire and sometimes yearn to look like these celebrities. I understand this, but these beautiful young women are made up for the entertainment world—they do not live your lifestyle.

Eye Beauty Workshop

Six teenage participants shared their eye problems with me, which I evaluated and then recommended a course of action. Please observe the following photographs and beauty comments.

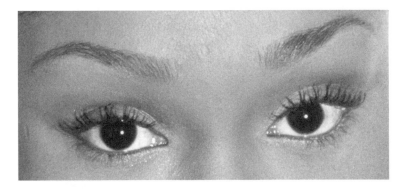

This is the perfect eye shape, with just the right space between the eyelid and brow. Brush and shape your brows. To be creative, highlight the brow bone with an ivory shadow. Contour the center of the eye with a deep rich brown and deep brassy gold on the lid and blend both colors form top to bottom. A rich brown eyeliner is then applied with matching lash-lengthening mascara.

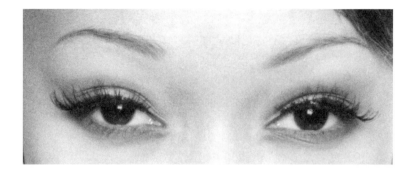

The lashes displayed here are too long, look artificial, and age your young eyes. For fun, though, they can be an evening effort! For day, however, I suggest a short or demi-length fake lash or none at all. Eyeliner should start deep in the inner corner of the eyelid, extending to the outer corner of the eye, moving toward the temple area. Use soft brown-black or soft black matte eyeliner on both upper and lower lids, and rich lash-building mascara for lower lashes. If your brows are too thin, as shown here, use a pencil to fill in. More brow hair from the bridge of the nose to the center of the brow arch would bring more balance and is more fashionable.

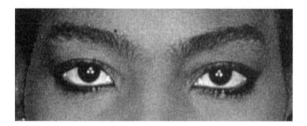

Bad shaping and overtweezed brows emphasize protruding eyes. The goal here should be to deemphasize the puffy part of the eyelid. The brow falls too deep into the corner of the eye. It should be a bit higher, and the arch should peak off the center of the pupil, moving outward toward the temples. (Tweezing is suggested here.) A powder brow formula can be brushed on the brows to give them a fuller, healthier look until the natural hairs grow back in. Subtle, muted shades should be applied on the puffy part of the eyelid and the prominent fashion color below it. Matching eyeliner is recommended, with an application of rich-toned mascara on the lashes.

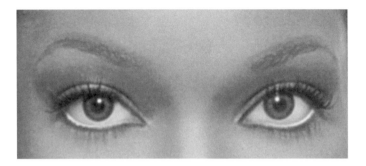

These are lovely eyes with great brows that frame the area with style. I recommend a rich brown brush-on-brow powder formula for slightly more brow definition. Use subtle, muted, no-sheen colors for daytime, with deep colors applied on the lid up to the crease for a contour. Avoid frosty, high sheen or shiny highlight colors on the brow bone.

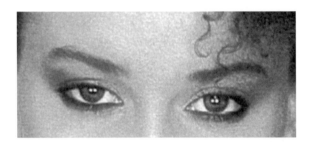

The primary goal here is to open your eyes, so brow maintenance and shaping are a must. Following these steps, add eyebrow and color prominence: first, highlight the brow bone with a high sheen or bright color. Then contour the crease of the eyelid with a darker color, and finally, apply intense coloring on the eyelid next to the lash, followed by lash-thickening mascara.

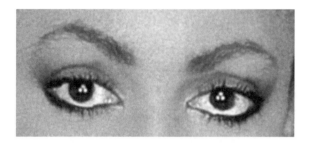

If you have thick and wide brows, as displayed here, I suggest that you go to a full-service beauty salon that specializes in brow care. Tweezing is best for teenagers. Ask questions and find out how you can copy the professional techniques at home for those in-between touch-ups. Keep in mind that when your brows are being shaped, the brow line should begin slightly in from the inner corner of the eye, and the arch should peak just beyond the center of the eye, with the brow ending slightly beyond the outer corner of the eye. To enhance your eyes even more, apply a kohl brown shadow on the thickest part of your eyelid, ending near the brow bone. Then use a bright complementary highlighter near the brow, blending the two colors where they meet. Finally, apply a bronze or gold shade at the lower part of the lid and blend with the other shades. Add eyeliner and mascara for a perfect ending.

TEEN TIP

The best suggestion that I could offer a teenage girl regarding her personal beauty regimen is: wear makeup that looks natural and that is appropriate for your age group.

—SYNCHANA
Harlem, New York, age 16

Be certain, the eyes have it!

For teenagers who live traditional lifestyles, too much makeup on dark eyelids is unattractive. Never overdo your eyes. I will show you how to make sure that everything blends and nothing is overstated, even if you add a little pizzazz for your very special occasions. Now, let's begin to dress your eyes with appropriate color.

How to Apply Eye Makeup

I have designed a simple system for you. It is a four-step, full-scale rainbow eye system in which we consider the correct approach to the eye shape, eyeliner, and lash application. The color chart in the middle of the book will guide you in making appropriate color choices. The major principle is to keep the look clean, blended, and subtle. The exception is with evening makeup, when you should exaggerate to shine and sparkle, when pizzazz is the operative word. Here is the order for applying eye makeup:

Steps for Applying Eye Makeup

1 Eyebrow makeup

2 Eyeliner

3 Eye shadow

4 Mascara

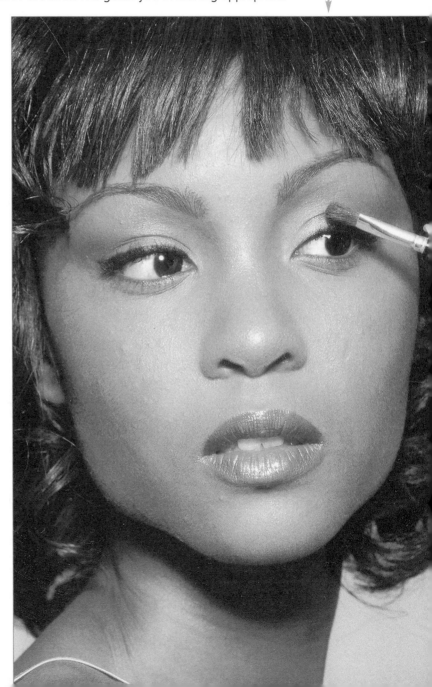

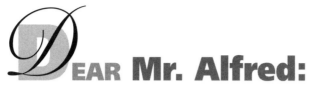

EAR Mr. Alfred:

What are some of the pros and cons of arching your eyebrows when you are trying to go for the natural look?

—GENNA
Montclair, New Jersey, age 14

Dear Genna:

I find it most unattractive when a teen shaves off her eyebrows and then uses an eyebrow pencil to draw in a line. This gives your face a severe look. So don't shave the eyebrow off and then put a new one on. Instead, shape or fill in your existing eyebrow.

—MR. ALFRED

Eyebrow Grooming

Blessed is the teen who does not have gaps and scars in her eyebrows. You are considered lucky if you have eyebrow hairs that lie flat and eyebrows that are well shaped to complement your eyes. You will not need eyebrow makeup. If you are one of these teens, then all you have to do is groom and shape your eyebrows with a brush.

For those of you who have thin eyebrows, an eyebrow pencil can fill in the spaces among the hairs and cover any scarring in the brow area. If you have unruly eyebrows, though, let's take care of that right now. Bushy or heavy and coarse eyebrows may require some plucking, and knowing the technique of how to shape your eyebrows is very important.

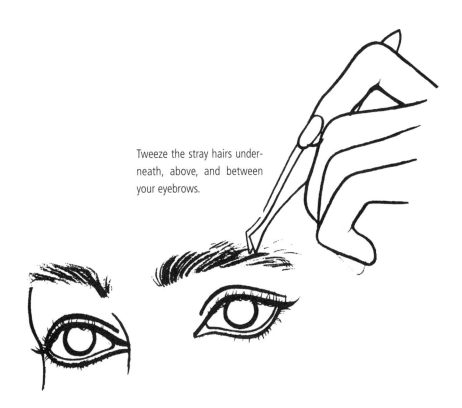

Tweeze the stray hairs underneath, above, and between your eyebrows.

Reshaping Your Eyebrows? Here's How

Step One   Brush brow upward, moving from the center of your forehead toward the temple area—trimming away unwanted individual hairs—following the pencil guide line. Relax and take your time. Brush hairs back in place.

Step Two   Still too full and bushy?
Brush hairs downward with the brow brush and move from the center of the bridge of the nose outward to the temple area. This second observation should reveal a more groomed appearance. Brush hairs back into place.

Step Three   Trim away protruding hairs.
Use eye makeup remover to wipe away traces of pencil guideline. Do you have a few spaces in your brow from missing hairs? Fill in with complementary brow pencil, or create a little drama with brush-on-brow powder for evening.

Nothing is more unsightly than a dramatic, overplucked eyebrow. The problem that this may cause—beyond unsightliness—is that when you continually pluck hairs in certain spots, you pull out some of the roots, and the hairs will never grow back. Thus you are left with a patchy-looking brow. So please be careful. You might prefer to leave eyebrow shaping to a professional.

If you opt to do it yourself, look in the mirror and honestly assess the length and thickness of your brows. If they are bushy and overpower your face, then you should remove some hairs. To tweeze an eyebrow, start from the center of its eye and go upward to the temple, removing from eight to ten hairs. Tweeze the stray hairs underneath your brow also. If your eyebrows are too thick and spotty with nicks, then you should shape the brow to complement a natural eyebrow line. With a brow pencil or powder and brow brush, you can stroke in between the spaces, filling and shaping the brow.

REVIEW!

1 The ideal eyebrow arch is smooth and soft—often referred to as a moon shape.

2 Shape your eyebrow with the peak at the top of your pencil in the center of the brow.

3 Eyebrows can easily be filled in with a pencil to give more definition to the line.

4 Eyebrow makeup can also be used where you have overtweezed or overplucked.

5 Shape the eyebrow with the pencil and fill in until new growth appears, then do your reshaping.

Determining Eyebrow Length

To determine the best length and thickness of your brow, hold the pencil to each nostril and straight up along the nose to the eyebrow. Where it touches the eyebrow is where the brow should begin. Hair between the eyebrows should be removed. Position the pencil vertically over the center of your eye to the beginning of the arch. When you position the pencil from the nose to the outer edge of the eye, you determine the endpoint of the brow and arch.

Don't be afraid to experiment with the eyebrow. Some eyebrows look great brushed straight up, toward the hairline; just brush them up and fan them out toward the temples. This is a great look, especially for evening.

Eyeliner Essentials

Eyeliners come in formulas designed for each skin type and in different forms: soft pencil, liquid, cream, and pressed cake.

Eyeliners are used to give more definition to the eyes. They highlight the eyes and make the eyelashes appear fuller and thicker. A person can really bring the desired effect to the eyes with a liner; it is the ultimate groomer because it separates the shadow from the lashes via a circle around the eyes.

I think the complementary neutral tones are most attractive on black teens. When you use eyeliner, be sure to color the top lid as well as the bottom.

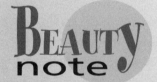

BEAU**T**Y
note

Are you having difficulty finding an eyeliner to complement your various shades of eye shadow or your pupils? If so, take your eye shadow color—maybe the corresponding shade in a dual kit—and simply wet your brush, then stroke the cake of eye shadow to create your eyeliner color. For example, if you want to use a brownish eye shadow close to the lash, with a dominant brown eyeliner, moisten your brush and then stroke with the brown shadow; draw in the color and, presto, you have an eyeliner in a corresponding shade.

Pencil versus Liquid Eyeliners

Liquid eyeliner is still one of the most popular forms, but I recommend the pencil eyeliner because you can control it better. Pencils come in more colors, they can be smudged on the top and bottom of the eyelids, and they can be applied either thick or

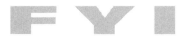

thin. If you have had very little practice applying liquid eyeliner, you can easily lose control. Yet both forms are serviceable and can produce attractive results.

Purchasing Your Eyeliner

The eyeliner should be color coordinated with your eye shadow. Eyeliners, especially pencils, can be tested at the cosmetics counter. Testing foundations as well as eye, cheek, and lip colors is permitted in department stores, chain stores, and some pharmacies. And you should test the colors. Try to test them in natural light, even if you have to stroke the color on your face or eyelid and then excuse yourself to walk to where there is natural light. Use your makeup mirror to look at the color on your skin. You will see that in different lighting the shades appear differently.

Here are a few words of caution. There are waterproof eyeliners that tend to be a little rubbery, but they are excellent if you perspire heavily, if your skin is oily, or if you go swimming a lot. However, I have found that when used frequently these waterproof eyeliners can actually dry out the area around your eyes, leaving it sensitive. This is especially true for those who suffer from allergies or who are naturally sensitive in this area. If this describes you, then I suggest you avoid the waterproof eyeliners.

SMART *and* SENSIBLE SUGGESTIONS FOR YOU
Annoying Allergies

According to Dr. Susan Taylor, "There are a host of various cosmetics with different ingredients. If a teen experiences itching or redness, or bumps, from her makeup, then use of that makeup should be discontinued immediately. You should not try another makeup until the rash symptoms resolve completely. Then you can read the list of ingredients and find a different makeup type that does not have that ingredient in it.

An allergy is a reaction of the body to a foreign material that it tries to reject or forms a reaction to it. Allergies can come from various foods, particularly shellfish and nuts. In terms of cosmetics, allergies can come from hair dyes, particularly black hair dyes that contain a chemical, para phenylenediamine, that commonly causes allergies. Nail polishes and lacquers contain formaldehydes that can cause allergic reactions not only on the hands, but particularly around the eyes. Eyeliner, mascara, and contact lens solutions all can cause allergies of the skin."

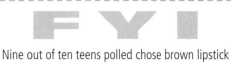

Eye-Catching Eye Shadow

The most popular eye shadows come in cream, crayon, and powder. The cream shadows are applied with an eye shadow sponge or your fingertip. This is best for teens with very dry eyelids. The crayon shadows are excellent for smoothing on and blending in. They can be very soft, and that is the caution for those of you who have oily skin. Make sure you don't overuse an oil-based crayon shadow, for it can build up a crease and melt on the eyelids. Powder shadows are applied with an eye shadow brush or sponge. They are ideal for most skin types because they can be controlled easily and they appear to be softer, silkier, and smoother on your skin. However, the powders are best suited for oily, combination, and normal to oily skin.

There are several cosmetics companies that encourage customers to dampen their powder eye shadows because it gives it a different consistency and helps them glide on evenly, dry well, and stay put. The color remains true and stays put, without the creasing so often seen when a cream shadow is used. This technique is excellent for oily skin.

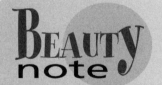
There are also fragrance-free eye shadows for those of you who have sensitive eyes or tend to have an allergy-prone eye area.

Eye shadows can be purchased separately or in multicolor kits. Many companies sell eye shadows that are sold as dual kits: two pans containing two colors that usually are a highlighter and a fashion shade, which can also be used for contours. There are also four-pan color kits: highlighter, contour, and a fashion shade in a light and a dark hue, and even six- and twelve-color pan kits that permit you to mix and blend shades to come up with original colors for a rainbow eye, smoldering eye, or contour eye.

Contour shades usually come in neutral colors like cocoa or light brown, or in shades

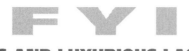

LONG AND LUXURIOUS LASHES

Your curly lashes look thick and luxurious. If you don't have enough curl, here's how you get it. Look directly into a mirror. Take the lash curler, open it, and bring it right up toward your eye. Secure your lashes between the rubber grips and squeeze for about fifteen seconds. *Voilà!* Curly lashes, ready to coat with your favorite color mascara!

of gray and in the berry shades. Highlighters do not have to be eggshell white or creamy white. They can be pink or dark lavender, or a light shade of blue, or even a dark shade of blue. The highlighter you use depends on the effect you want. Experiment to come up with original ideas, but consult my color chart for your best colors.

When applying mascara to curly lashes, brush from the top of the lash down first; then from the bottom up.

Mascara

The purpose of mascara is to build up your lashes. Mascara makes your lashes look longer, thicker, and more smoldering. There is a formulation that comes as a cream, which I recommend.

The shades that look best on black teens are black, brown-black, dark brown, antique bronze, and berry shades, the newest entries on the market. Don't be turned off by the color intensity in the tube. When applied, these berry shades look very soft around the eyes. In fact, the raspberry, cranberry, green, and navy blue shades look fabulous! Pay attention to your mix of colors when you make up, though. Be careful what color eye shadow you use with a colored mascara. Coordinate the colors between the lashes and the eyelid itself.

SMART *and* SENSIBLE SUGGESTIONS FOR YOU

If you want to test a mascara before you buy it, don't allow the beauty adviser to apply it from the tester wand directly to your eyelashes. Bacteria grows extremely fast in the dark, warm tubes on the lighted cosmetics counter, and that tester wand could put bacteria in your eyes, so make sure you get a clean wand.

Blushers for a Special Glow

The purpose of a blusher is to bring a blush and glow to the cheeks. I recommend using blushers because they bring a vibrancy and a live quality to your face. But you must carefully select the color and place it correctly.

Don't be dissuaded from using blusher because you see intense color compacts on display at retail cosmetics counters. They are usually very bright or very intense, but you will be surprised how, when keyed to your skin color, those deep, rich, pigmented blushers bring a soft natural glow to your cheeks.

You have probably heard the cosmetics trade call their blusher colors Mahogany, Golden Bronze, Loganberry, Raspberry, Topaz, Ruby, Ginger, Gold, Cinnamon, and Brown. These are the names of just a few of the blusher products produced. Several companies have developed many natural, warm, and sophisticated deep-pigmented shades for black skin that have proved to be excellent.

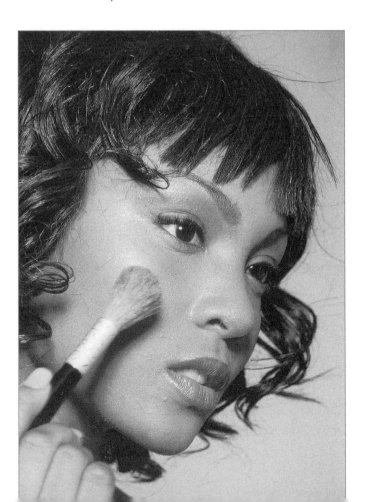

Your lipstick and blusher do not have to match; however, they should be of the same color family or in the same color range. For example, a red-brown blusher enhances a yellow-based red lipstick. For special occasions, a true red blusher with golden highlights makes a wonderful partner to a gold-frosted red lipstick with a golden gloss. With this combination, your cheeks and lips will be all aglow with golden sparkle, reflecting light against your dark skin.

Many kinds of blushers are sold that produce different effects and are designed for different skin types. The two major types are: powders and creams.

Powder Blushers

Powder imparts a natural-looking, soft matte finish. Of all the formulas, it is the easiest to apply and looks the best on black skin. Powders glide on smoothly and don't leave a bumpy, ashen buildup. Literally hundreds of powder blushers are available, tailored for every skin type. If you try a blusher that gives a gray appearance to your skin, you can be sure it was not designed for your skin coloring. All skin types can wear powder blusher; however, they are best for those with combination or oily skin. Teens with sensitive skin must be very careful and only use blushers designed for sensitive skin.

Cream Blushers

There are two basic cream blushers—regular and oil free—and they come as a swivel stick or in a compact. Use your fingers or the swivel stick for best application. Apply the cream over your foundation and then add your translucent powder. In general, cream blushers are easy to blend, but avoid the pale shades, red to pinks, and peachy to orange colors, because they appear to be suspended in air or to sit on top of the skin.

Cream blushers are best for combination or dry skin. Oily skin collects the shine and high humidity, and in summer months the cheeks appear greasy and slick—not attractive at all! All skin types should stay away from the frosted cream blushers unless the frost is gold, not silver. I don't think silver enhances medium to dark complexions, and it should never be used on the cheeks.

Types of Blushers

1 *Gel tint.* Gives a nice translucent finish. Less is best. Good for combination to oily skin (most are oil free and water based); not advised for very dry skin; can appear

shiny and slick. To apply, use fingertips, on top of foundation, before powder; dry-down period is extremely fast, so you have to work quickly; gel can streak and blotch

2 *Liquid.* This is moist and smooth and good for all skin types; it is best suited for combination, medium to dry skin. To apply, use a sponge, sliding on top of foundation, then set with powder; easy to apply.

3 *Mousse.* Soft and dewy looking, this is not for dry skin but for oily or combination skin. To apply, use fingertips; blend with a sponge, especially around the edges.

4 *Cream.* Soft and dewy looking, this is best with no foundation. It is good for normal to dry skin; oil free is best suited for only those with oily skin. To apply, use fingertips and blend on top of foundation; set with powder.

5 *Powder.* Use this to create a matte or semimatte frost (for special occasions). Though good for all skin types, it is especially beneficial for oily skin. To apply, use a blush brush.

Use Blushers with Moderation

The ideal application should create only a suggestion, or hint, of color. Select rich, pure colors such as copper-bronze with its deep gold base, or a soft plum, light wine-burgundy, or a deeply pigmented almond-orange shade. When you apply powder blusher, always dip the brush quickly and flick or twist your wrist to stroke the cheek lightly. Remember: it is better to apply just a little blusher and then go back and apply more if you need it, than to apply too much and have to disturb the foundation to remove the excess. Matte colors (no shine) are best for day on all skin types.

Color Placement

The cheek, according to your facial shape and size, is where you should place the blusher. Don't place it on the nose. After all, why put blusher where it will make you look like you have a cold?

The outer corner of your eye is your guideline for application. Don't ever bring the color toward the broad nostril of your nose; it will broaden your facial structure. Likewise, blusher should not ever be shaded down past the tip of your nose. Draw an imaginary line from the tip of your nose, under your natural cheekbone, to the middle part of

Special Stuff

Blushers can do more to add warmth and radiance than any other cosmetics. For the ultimate, long-lasting glow, apply a cream blusher over your foundation and set it with translucent powder. Then apply a complementary powder blusher over the translucent face powder and blend. You will have a day-long natural glow.

your ear; this is usually where you should cut off the shading. Don't apply blusher too close to the eyes—it can make them look puffy and drawn.

Do You Know Your Face Shape?

Contouring or shading your facial features is the easiest way to slim down the face and redefine flawed features.

We feature the following four basic face shapes; however, different faces require different techniques. If your face shape is not here, combine the features from others to obtain the right techniques.

To find your face shape, tie your hair up and away from your face and look into the mirror. If you still can't tell, get a ruler and measure your forehead from temple to tem-

ple, cheekbone to cheekbone, and jawline to jawline. Place these measurements on a piece of paper and connect with rounded lines.

Square Face

You have a firm structure, usually a wide forehead, cheeks, and jawline. The apple, or round part of the cheekbone, registers near the outer corner of your eye. Begin the blusher application at this point, sweeping the cheek color upward to the center part of the ear. To soften a wide and square face, apply cheek color at the bottom side of the jaw, with the cheekbone to accent the center of your face. Don't ever apply blusher between the "no blush zone" apple of the cheekbone and the bloom of the nostril.

Your eyebrows are most important and should never be straight thin lines. Looking straight into the mirror, arch your brows at the corner of the pupil, so they are in line with your cheekbones.

Round Face

You have a solid, structured face. Keep color high on the cheekbones, sweeping it outward and upward to the top of the ear and hairline. Don't ever place color on the apple and never bring color from the apple toward the bloom of the nose. Sweep blusher from the outer corner of the eye, fanning upward. The eyes are the focal point.

Eyebrows should be naturally full and shaped horizontally, with a slight curve. Keep lip pencil line faint and inside the natural lip line.

Oval Face

You have the so-called balanced facial structure. Polish the cheekbone with rich radiant color, sweeping from the outer edge of the corner of your eye and creating a V effect. The open part of the V spreads wide toward the ear and hairline. Play up the apple, moving straight across and

Special Blusher Notes

- Apply radiant, vibrant blusher with your brush sweeping across the cheekbone, blending upward to the top of the ear.
- Use your contour brush and apply a rich matte brown on the bottom side of your cheekbone, moving upward toward the center part of your ear.
- For that special glow at night, apply flesh-toned golden powder blusher on temples, between the eyes, on the tip of your nose, and at the base of your chin.
- To deemphasize a full or square chin, use your contour brush with a matte brown blusher.

fanning outward. Place shading color at the temples, on the tip of the nose, and at the chin. Lips are shaped, moist, and dewy.

Eyebrows take on a subtle half-moon shape. Accentuate the crease and create a more concave illusion. Highlight with mascara.

Oblong

You have a slim, delicate structure. Start your blusher placement at the outer edge of the apple. Keep color on the cheekbone, toward the top. Make wide sweeps toward the upper part of your ear and hairline. You want to create optical and esthetic horizontal lines of color to suggest width. Don't shade or contour the temples, jawline, or chin. Color in the center zone of the face is important.

Eyebrows should be on a horizontal plane, with a high center arch. Eye shadow is earthy, gold, topaz, peachy-red, soft berry, no brown-black or black outer corner shading. Lip pencil liner should emphasize, broaden, and play up full lips. Apply color to the very edge.

Your Fabulous Lips

The Beauty of Full Lips

I feel that the most attractive feature of an African American teenager's face is her lips. No one smiles with such full lips and with such beautiful white teeth. The maturing black female teenager who believes that black is really beautiful has no problem accepting God's gift.

Your lips dramatically outline your mouth. Therefore, your teeth must not be a major negative to an otherwise beautiful face. When you have moist, dewy, luscious lips, your white and even teeth make you even more inviting, and your smile will make your face radiant, bringing joy to all those who see you.

Lip Shape and Appearance

You shape, contour, and tone your body, and you must also strengthen lip muscles by toning and shaping them. Believe it or not, smiling will maximize the value and beauty of your lips. Learn how to express your lovely features by practicing different looks before a mirror. If your bottom lip hangs down or if your lips have droopy, turned-down corners (you look sad to others), you must teach yourself to lift the corners up.

In addition to how you hold your lips, your mouth may have other "spoilers" needing attention. For example, missing teeth, gold teeth on a girl (please), yellow teeth, or poorly manufactured and installed braces (the different colors or clear and invisible are fabulous choices). Mouth odor is definitely out. (Use mouthwash and talk to your dentist if this problem persists.) Our ancestors would chew "sweet leaves" like parsley and spearmint to take care of that condition. Chapped, cracked, peeling, or bleeding lips on anyone is unattractive. (Use lip lubricants and moisturizers if this is your problem.)

Glorious Lips

Brilliant colors on light-to-dark skin are fabulous. Usually, though, they are not recommended for daytime activities. Red, for example, is a great shade, but the wrong red just looks awful! Some come with yellow- and blue-based overtones, so always try before you buy.

The following three lip illustrations define the strength of the lip line, shading, and confirming the lip color. Study all three looks and compare their physical composition to yours.

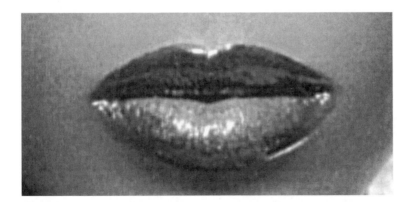

Here, the bow of the top lip is firm and nicely contrasted by the pout in the center of the plump bottom lip. If the top lip is darker than the bottom lip, you can use lip toners, balancers, and lip-lightening correctors to reflect light and stain pink discolorations, thereby creating an even tone. Set the lips with translucent powder and apply lipstick color and gloss.

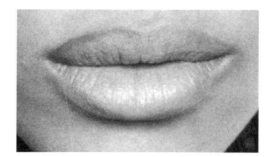

What a gorgeous look for a teenager! This is an excellent example of daytime lip color. Sheer lip toners and lipstick give the illusion of less, which is often best. The lips are softly concaved with a purring pout, giving an impression of innocence.

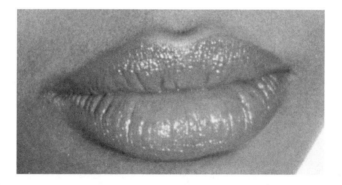

The natural V-bowed lips were dressed with blended colors that complement the skin tone. A lip brush was used to apply color in the recessed grooved areas to produce a smooth, supple, and soft appearance. Color, which was applied directly from the tube, glides over the grooves. You have it, girl—smooth and supple lips, sought after in Hollywood!

Maximize the value and beauty of your fabulous lips and learn how to express your natural charm. Stand in front of a mirror and smile. Your lips, teeth, and smile will make your face radiant, bringing joy to you and all who see you.

Lip Color Options

You might wish to apply a lipstick product from a tube, crayon, wand, pan, or pot or use a lip brush. There are great clear lip glosses and lip moisturizers that impart a moist sheer sheen to your lips. They can be worn alone, or if you prefer, with just a hint of natural color. Try lipsticks in earth tones to soft beige, or pink tones. You might want to take the time to use a lip pencil, which is an excellent tool for achieving a natural look. If you use a lip pencil, lightly line the lip and fill in with the pencil, covering any uneven tones, then apply a clear red, a brown lip shade, or clear tint gloss. However, avoid using greasy, nonpenetrating petroleum jelly—it looks and feels tacky on your lips.

For those of you who prefer rich lip color, I recommend deep orange shades such as Cinnamon-Orange, Burnt Orange, Radiant Red, Bronze-Coral, and Claret.

Lipstick Tools

Now let's see how to use the various lipstick tools and materials: lip liner pencil, lip brush, lip light, lip toner or foundation, and lip balancer.

1 *Lip liner pencil.* Liner pencils define the line of the lips and should be chosen with your skin tone in mind. For example, if you have fair to light skin, your liner should be rose-pink, light red, light plum, or light brown. Teens with medium skin tones look best when they use liner pencils in shades of red, light brown, brown, and plum. Those with dark skin tones look best using red, deep brown, raspberry, plum, or brown-black liners. Never use a black pencil to line your lips. It's unattractive and appears harsh.

When you want a new look for your lips, use a lip pencil to outline it. Lightly outline the lips and fill in the corners if your lips are full, and then edge in your selected color. The pencil should match as closely as possible the desired lip color.

The lip liner pencil also keeps lip color from bleeding and gives a more precise lip line. When matte, oil-free pencils are used as a base for cream or frosted lipsticks, the color stays put and wears much longer.

2 *Lip brush.* The purpose of a lipstick brush is to transfer lipstick from the tube to the surface of the lips. The lip brush gets color into the crevices, giving a smooth, full-color application; and it also gives you the option of lining your lips, reducing the possibility of your lipstick bleeding once the large area is colored.

A lipstick brush may be either man-made, of natural fibers, or a combination of both. I prefer a blend of natural and man-made fibers.

3 *Lip light.* Lip light is a lip color adjuster, which reflects light colors away from ruddy, bluish, or very dark lips; it is worn under the lipstick.

4 *Lip toner.* A lip toner, or foundation, is a lip adjuster that corrects slightly discolored lips, evens out lip tones, and keeps color true. Toners come in fair-to-medium and medium-to-dark shades.

5 *Lip balancer.* A lip balancer is a deep, waxy, purplish teak natural pigment, designed to camouflage the resistant light pink discoloration often found on medium and dark lips. A lip balancer also neutralizes the acidity that causes discoloration in the center of the bottom lip, an area that is more often affected than the upper. In the process, it prevents the lipstick from changing color when placed on this area. A lip balancer is worn under the lipstick. It is excellent for subtle, medium, and deep shades of lipstick; however, the bright reds, orange-browns, and light berry shades are affected by a lip balancer.

Types of Lipstick

Choosing a lipstick is a very personal preference, so it is up to you to select the ones you like best. Lipsticks with specially formulated conditioners, moisturizers, waxes, and light mineral oil are superior to those without them, since these ingredients smooth the lips, help retain moisture, help prevent infection, and often protect sensitive skin.

Here's a special beauty note: most lipstick formulas include conditioners and emollients. For example, lip moisturizers often contain PABA (a sunscreen) along with vitamins A and E. So there are advantages over and above beauty for using a lipstick.

Now, let's review some of the major types of lipstick available today:

1 *Cream lipsticks.* Standard cream lipsticks are deep pigment colors without shine. They wear longer and impart more coverage than the noncream sticks, owing to their heavy wax base. A second cream formula is more lightweight in texture and does not feel as heavy on the lips, but it also does not wear as long because it usually has a mineral-oil base.

2 *Frosted lipsticks.* Frosted lipsticks are usually heavy pigment colors with an iridescent, pearlized, or opaque gold coverage. Black teens look best wearing lipsticks with a gold or yellow base.

3 *Silver-sparkling frost.* I don't recommend silver-sparkling frosts because they impart an ashy gray look to red-brown or bluish-brown skin undertones.

4 *Long-lasting lipsticks.* New research and development has produced long-wearing, nonsmear lipstick formulas.

5 *Matte lipsticks.* No-shine lipstick formulas have conditioners for a nondry look and feel.

6 *Translucent lipsticks.* Translucent lipsticks in tubes or wands impart just a hint of color, with sheer coverage.

7 *Lip glosses.* Glosses have a clear, shiny, transparent base. They come in pans, pots, wands, and tubes. Some have conditioners and moisturizers, and claim healing properties. They are usually worn over lipstick to impart a sheer gloss. Lip glosses can be worn alone, as well.

8 *Nonfragrance lipsticks.* Fragrance-free lipsticks are for sensitive and acned skin. When some teens have an allergic swelling, or experience an itchy, burning sensation on their lips, they may be having an adverse reaction to their lipstick. Most teens sensitive to lipstick are reacting to the lanolin, fragrance, dyes, or preservatives in the formula. If this is a problem for you, buy fragrance-free, dermatologically tested, hypoallergenic lipstick.

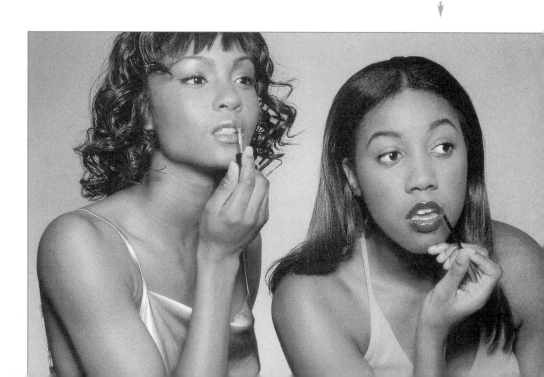

Applying Lip Color

The lip brush is used to pick up a small amount of lip color, and then to outline the lips, filling in from the center of the mouth to the outer edges. The following is the procedure I suggest for creating beautifully colored lips:

Steps for Coloring Your Lips

1 Apply a lip color adjuster, such as lip light (optional).

2 Outline your lips with a sharp lip liner pencil.

3 Edge in the lipstick color along the pencil outline and coat the lips, starting with the bottom and moving to the upper lip. Apply more color in the center, moving outward to the edges. If your lips are smooth, apply color directly from the tube.

4 Add lip gloss for a moist effect or gleam.

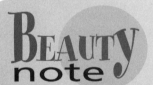

Love Your Lips

The dark upper lip is a beautiful contrast to the healthy pink bottom lip, or vice versa. Do what actresses and supermodels of color do: treat your lips as a beauty asset. Flaunt those full lips with plum, brown, mocha, cinnamon, or red lip liner pencil. Then apply clear or colored lip gloss, starting from the corners in toward the center of your lips. Presto!

Let's Review!! The Ultra-Grand Makeup Application

Here we suggest the appropriate makeup steps to maintain your warm, healthy youthful appeal.

Start with a clean, fresh face.

Step One—*Foundation* - - - - - - - ▶

Tool—*Makeup sponge*

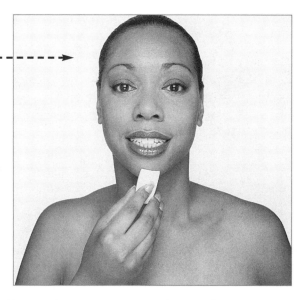

Concealer is applied to the entire eyelid to serve as a foundation for eye shadow (shadow stays in place longer and appears to be smoother) and undereye area to give a smoother effect and conceal uneven, blotchy skin tones. A damp sponge is preferred (a dry sponge lifts too much foundation). Place foundation on uneven parts of the face first and fill in. Blend and then observe. If necessary, cover the entire face. Final movement should be light, downward strokes. (Set your foundation with translucent powder. If your skin is very dry to extremely dry, powder is optional.)

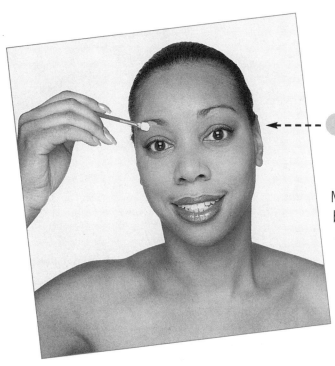

◀ - - - - - **Step Two**—*Eye shadow*

Tool—*Eye makeup applicator*

Movements—highlight brow bone. Contour center of eye to give the concave effect and finally apply the fashion color closet to the eyelash area. Blend and set with powder.

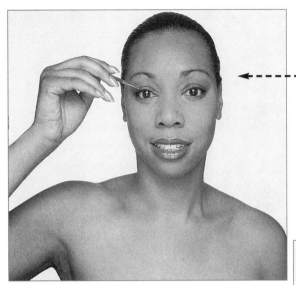

Step Three—*Eyeliner*

Tool—*Eyeliner pencil, liquid or cake powder liner*

Should be applied close to the lashes, drawing line from inner to outer corners.

Step Four—*Brows*

Tool—*Brow comb and brush, brow gel, cake powder brush-on-brow, and pencil*

Fill in brow spaces with brow pencil or cake powder and comb or brush back into shape. If hairs are unruly, apply brow gel. If gel is tinted, apply and brush.

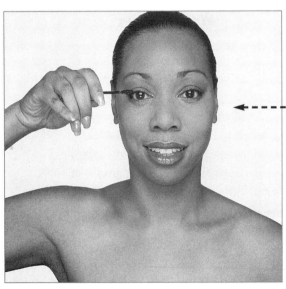

Step Five—*Eyelashes*

Tool—*Eyelash wand*

Apply lash-building, waterproof, or sensitive-formula mascara. Stroke up and out. If lashes are extremely curly, hold wand vertically, as demonstrated, and swing left to right, hitting the tips of the lashes.

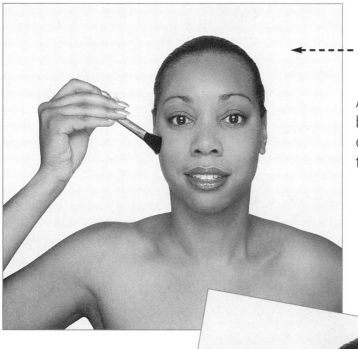

Step Six—*Blush*

Tool—*Blush brush*

Apply blush to cheek-bone area. Move along check area outward to the hairline.

Step Seven—*Lips*

Tool—*Lip brush, lip liner pencil, lip toner*

Apply lipstick with a brush to fill in the grooves or lines on lips or lip lines with lip liner for shaping, and color the discolored lip with pencil, and fill in with lip color and gloss.

QUIZ ADDING COLOR TO YOUR FACE

1
Q. Where do you start adding blusher?
A. Use the outer corner of your eye as a guide to start adding blusher.

2
Q. What skin type should use powder eye shadow?
A. Powder eye shadow is good for all skin types.

3
Q. What zone do you avoid when applying blusher?
A. Never apply blusher in the "no blush zone" between the apple of your cheekbone and the bloom of your nose.

4
Q. What should you do when you want to test mascara in the store?
A. Always ask the makeup artist for a clean wand to prevent the spread of bacteria.

5
Q. In which direction should you apply blusher?
A. Always move across, upward, and out toward the hairline.

6
Q. What lipstick shades would you wear to get a hint of natural color?
A. Try lipsticks in earth tones to soft beige or pink tones.

7
Q. Should you add blusher underneath your eyes?
A. No, do not add blusher underneath eyes near the lower rim.

8
Q. What is a matte color?
A. A color with no shine.

CHAPTER 4

Those Little Extras That Define You!

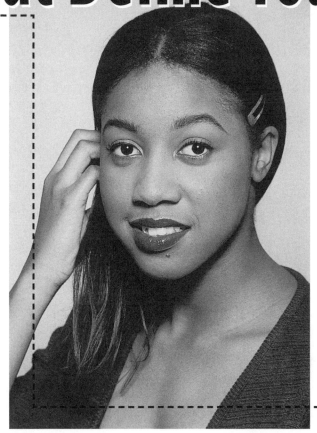

Y**OU'RE AN INDIVIDUAL.** All the little things you do and wear make you stand out and help create your own special identity. You want to look good! Feel good! Smell good! You know everybody wants to! Here's how!

Smellin' Good—Making Sense of Your Fragrance Choices

It's about pleasing the senses. Fragrances can be silent, suggestive, and should reveal something about your personality and your moods.

FYI

Don't fool yourself into thinking that fragrance will cover up body odor—it only intensifies it. Apply fragrance only to your fresh, clean skin.

Building Your Fragrance Collection

The average black teenager owns or purchases four to eight different scents. These purchases are made from the oil perfume vendors on the street, department stores, chains, drugstores, mail order, and of course through the Internet.

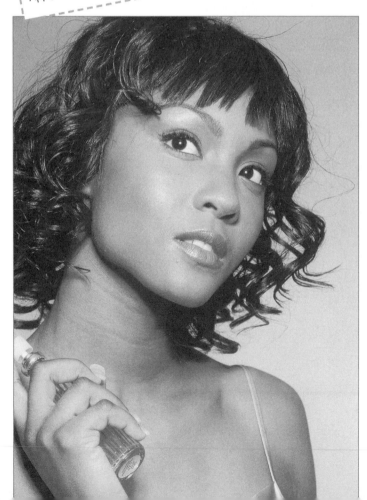

No matter how you purchase it, you must take some time to select a scent. Some teenagers like to have a scent arrive before they do and the essence of that scent linger after the grand departure. Some boys like girls who really smell good. Certain fragrances evoke past, present, and future. Some of your girlfriends like the silent, understated, but suggestive scents with an edge. Do you know what scent brings out your beauty and allure?

Consider your body's chemistry. What smells great on your girlfriends and seems just right may not produce the same effect on you and others. Fragrance develops differently on individual skin types, depending on natural skin oils, body temperature, and the season. If your skin is oily and the weather is hot, and you have selected an intense perfume, it evaporates faster, so the scent smells much stronger! If your skin is dry, and the fragrance is alcohol based, the fragrance sinks into the skin. You may have to reapply the fragrance several times to keep the scent potent.

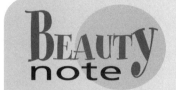

Fragrances are designed to mature on the skin at sensual spots.

Categories of Scent

- Floral is the power of one flower. The essence of gardenia is one fine example. Other elements support the top, middle, and bottom role of the fragrance.

- Modern blends of flowers are called florals. Synthetic scents match and support one another in this complex combination.

- Mossy green, reminiscent of a woodsy, outdoor autumn day, with combinations of ferns and herbs.

- Oriental scents are mysterious, sultry, and exotic. They denote luxury and opulence. Some blends include musk, patchouli, and sandalwood.

- Spicy includes extracts of cinnamon, vanilla, ginger, carnation, and cloves—the scent that tarries and hangs around. It evokes fond memories. One who can be sentimental, wishful, and regretful.

- Fruity fragrances are refreshing and light citrus blends. This happy-mood scent includes bits of lemon, mandarin, and lime.

  Top Note: First smell of the scent is called the top note.

  Middle Note: The main body of the fragrance. For example, woodsy, floral, Oriental, other.

  Bottom Note: The true essence of the scent, which lingers the longest, augmented by other aromatic blends.

Fragrance Classification

- Perfume is the longest-lasting concentrated form of fragrance.

- Perfume Solid Formula is one of the hottest concentrations that comes in a pot, solid cream, and a cream-to-powder compact.

- Perfume Oil is another hot and popular concentration with black teenagers. It's a real bargain when purchased from a street vendor who specializes in pure oil-based roll-on musk, for example.

- Eau de Parfum is a less concentrated form of full-strength perfume.

- Eau de Toilette is third in perfume intensity. It's excellent as an allover body splash or spray.

- Cologne is the lightest and most subtle form of perfume, and has less strength than eau de toilette.

- Splash and Mist or Eau Fraîche are the refreshing and lightest forms of fragrances. They are excellent as an aftershower or afterbath allover body splash or mist. Most are alcohol free. They are great for school, sport, and quick travel touch-ups.

How to Test a Fragrance

Apply fragrance to the underside of your wrist. For dry skin types, wait five minutes, and for oily skin types, wait ten minutes to discern the middle note. Remember, it is not the initial sniff that you are evaluating. After the other elements have evaporated, move away from the perfumed area of the cosmetics counter. Now, take a good long sniff of the wrist with the applied fragrance, and if it smells good, make your choice. If there is the slightest tinge of bad odor, you should reconsider.

Fragrance in Your Life

After a stressing exam, part-time job, or sport or exercise workout, wouldn't it be nice to come into your room at home—or dorm, hotel, or night over at your girlfriend's house—enlivened with your favorite fragrance? Fragrance helps to create a relaxing atmosphere.

Home and Dorm Room

For special occasions, try the real thing—a bunch of fragrant live flowers! Set several potpourri-filled bowls by your bed, chest of drawers, bookshelves, computer desk, and windowsills for total fragrance meltdown. I would like to suggest the following: for your closet, bedroom, and bath, buy scented drawer liners.

Fragrance in the Home

- Closet. Scented sachets are still in!

- Home or dorm room. Spray scents from a can on baseboards, in corners, around doorjambs, and throw rugs. Place sachets or scented soaps in your underwear drawer.

- Bath. Keep scented soaps and potpourri in a basket, on display. Spray towel collections with the lightest fragrance formulas.

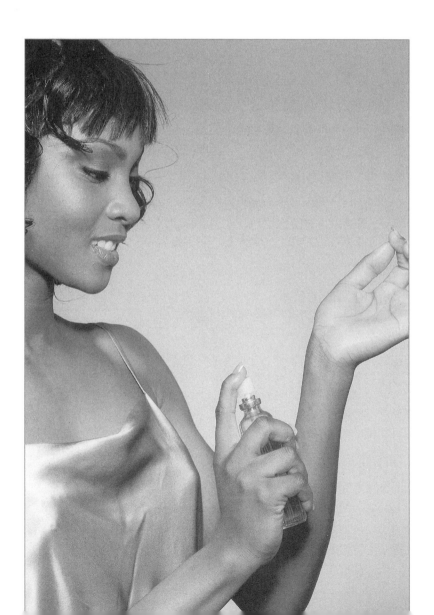

The Scented Bath

The bath can be the ultimate, inexpensive way to relax and emerge energized, invigorated, feeling lovely, relaxed, and free of tension. The bath experience can do all that and more!

Set the Mood

Start with soft music or environment mood sounds (try the sounds of a waterfall, ocean beach, or gentle stream), one or two scented candles, and a tall refreshing glass of your favorite flavored or mineral water. Now, draw warm tepid water (not hot), add bath oils or crystals, clear your mind, and then unwind and relax.

Now while you are relaxing, I would like to share with you some more soothing bath products for future in-bath experiences.

- *Dry-combination skin.* Bath oils add moisturizing emollients and lubricants.

- *Oily and troubled skin.* Bath gels are fine for those who miss soap. Gels clean the body gently and leave the body lightly scented and smooth.

- *All skin types.* Herbal bath beads impart all-natural conditioning care. A milk bath softens and silkens the body. Bubble bath contains emollients to relax and soften the skin. Scented crystals are heavily scented, and most add harmless colors to the water.

Your Tools for Bathing

- **Body Brush**
  Brings a nice healthy sheen to dark skin. Use a brush with natural bristles. Do not use rubber bath or synthetic bristles. (These bath tools will leave marks and cause uneven toned skin on most of us.)
- **Loofah**
  The loofah sloughs off dead skin cells, unclogs pores, softens and smooths the skin. Our ancestors have used this body bathing tool for centuries. It is the dried seedpod of a tropical gourd.
- **Other Bath Tools**
  The body cloth, friction mitt, and natural sea sponge are used for body cleansing and to help remove dead skin cells.

Let's now review and answer some of the most frequently asked questions about fragrances.

1   **Q.** Is one fragrance enough?
    A. Why not complement the many facets of your lifestyle? Spotlight these dimensions with a special scent. Build a collection so you will have a fragrance for every occasion.

2   **Q.** Which perfume will be right for me?
    A. Spray the fragrance on the underside of your wrist, wait about five to ten minutes, and then see how you like it. Make your choice.

3   **Q.** Where should I keep my perfume?
    A. Keep your perfume away from heat and direct sunlight. Always keep the cap on to prevent evaporation.

4   **Q.** What is the difference between perfume, cologne, and eau de toilette?
    A. Perfume is the most potent of all, eau do toilette is second in perfume intensity, and cologne is the lightest, most subtle form of fragrance.

5   **Q.** Does body chemistry affect fragrance?
    A. Whether you have oily, dry, or combination skin, the season of the year, the climate, and your body temperature all affect the performance of fragrance on your skin. Fragrances last longer on oily skin and in warm weather. In contrast, fragrance evaporates more rapidly on dry skin and in cold weather. No perfume smells exactly the same on two people.

*D*EAR **Mr. Alfred:**

One day after my mother left for work, I put on her per-fume and wore it to school. One day my friend asked me why was I wearing that "smelly stuff." My mother always gets compliments, how come I didn't?

—BARBARA
Baltimore, Maryland, age 15

Dear Barbara:

What smells good on your mom won't necessarily smell good on you. First of all, the fragrances she selects are for a more mature woman, and a fragrance develops differently on individual skin types and seldom smells the same on two people. Its reaction is based on natural skin oils, body temperature, and the seasons.

—MR. ALFRED

Now that we know all about smellin' good, let's take a look at our nails.

Basic Beauty Facts

For strong, healthy nails, a high-protein diet is best. It takes four to six months to grow a full-length new nail.

Your Glorious Nails—They Can Be Even More Beautiful!

Lovely hands can be the ultimate statement in your total grooming regimen. But making that statement requires proper care.

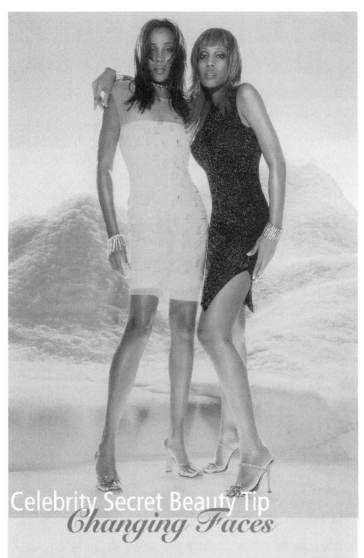

Celebrity Secret Beauty Tip
Changing Faces

To get the optimum look, we chose cutting-edge colors for our hair. They complement our skin tones, and with a little help from smoky gray shadows, bring attention to our eyes.

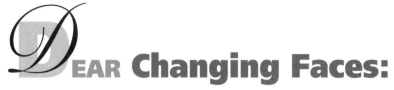

DEAR Changing Faces:

You have the most beautiful complexions. How do you find such natural makeup?

—DANISHA
Brooklyn, New York, age 17

Dear Danisha:

We are sticklers for a water regimen—eight glasses a day. We also have a routine of daily skincare—cleanse, tone, moisurize, and twice a month we have a professional salon facial treatment. With a smooth foundation, it's much easier to get makeup to look natural.

—CHANGING FACES

Hand Exam: Can You Positively Answer Yes To These Questions?

1 Are your nails uniformly shaped and proportionate lengths?

2 Are your nails healthy—minus splits and breaks?

3 Are your nails neatly manicured?

4 Are your knuckles soft and smooth?

5 Are your hands soft and supple on both the outer side and the palms?

Beautiful hands are the result of regular good care. If you find that your hands aren't as pleasing as they should be, the following will help you dramatically improve their overall appearance.

Your hands are constantly exposed to stresses: weather, pollutants, detergents and other irritating chemicals, and dirt. They get cut, bruised, and scraped. When you clean your hands, you usually wash them in soap and water, removing the limited moisture and oils the body provides to protect them. Your hands do not have as many oil-producing glands or as much fatty tissue per square inch as does your face. There are no oil glands on the palms of your hands (sweat glands, yes). Thus, washing with drying soaps is more stressful for your hands than you probably realize.

Ashen-colored skin between the thumb and index finger, and on the knuckles and cuticles, of black teens is an indication of poor hand care. Regardless of your skin tone, dry-looking skin is unattractive. It shows up more on dark skin, and therefore black skin requires a more intensive hand-care regimen. As you would suppose, the seasons of the year affect your hands differently; and the worst season is winter.

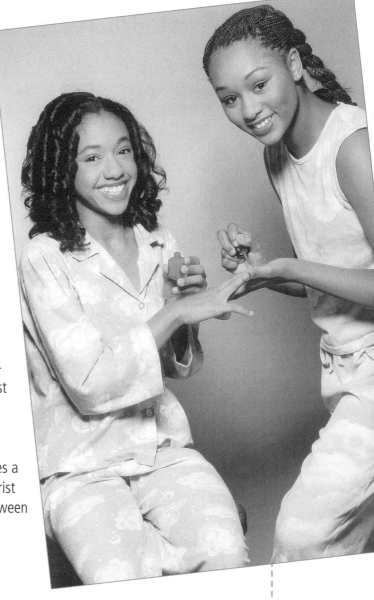

To care for your hands in winter, apply an extra-dry hand cream formula. I do not recommend petroleum jelly, since it gives the hands a greasy, tacky, dull look and feel. It also attracts dirt particles to the hands and under the nails, and it has no moisturizing or conditioning properties. There are excellent over-the-counter hand- and nail-care products to use, but you must use them regularly to achieve the best results.

Proper care for the hands also requires periodic, regular pampering, which includes a regular manicure. Learn from your manicurist how to care for your hands personally between visits.

Smart *and* Sensible Suggestions for You

- When you go to a manicurist, take your own tools with you. Buy everything and keep it in a little pouch. Then take it with you. This will help decrease the spread of infection.

- Artificial nails are fine for special occasions; you just don't want to wear them for long periods of time. If you're addicted to them, you need to take them off at least every three months or so and give your nails a rest. Prolonged use can lead to thinning of the nails and fungus and you can never regain your former strong nails.

—DR. SUSAN TAYLOR

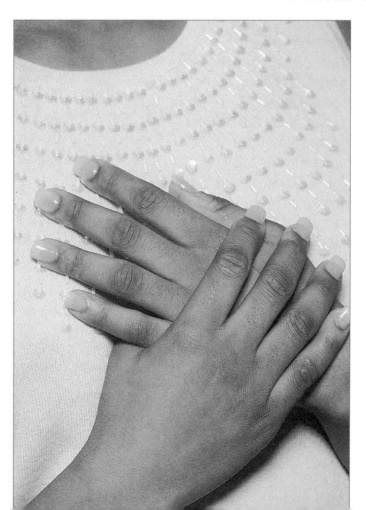

Nail Care

Parts of a Nail

Matrix—the formative intercellular tissue of the nail. Blood cells nourish the matrix.

Lunule—the whitish half-moon shape at the base of the fingernail.

Cuticle—a thin outer layer of the nail skin epidermis surrounding the nail.

Nail bed or plate—the part of your finger upon which the nail surface rests.

Manicure Tools

- Nail Polish Remover
- Cotton Balls and Pads
- Emery Board or Emery File
- Nail Soak
- Cuticle Lotion Remover
- Manicure Orange Stick or Cuticle Shaper
- Cuticle Trimmer
- Scissors
- Buffer
- Base Coat
- Nail Polish
- Clear Top Coat
- Quick-Drying or Speed-Drying Spray

COLOR SENSE

When choosing nail polish colors, remember that clear or neutral shades don't show up chips as much as darker or brighter colors. The lighter your polish, the longer your nails look. Shimmery, sparkly nail polish is great, but all your nail flaws will show.

The Basic Manicure—Ten Steps to Fabulous Nails

Step One. Start clean. Wash your hands. Wipe away all polish with an acetone-type polish remover.

Step Two. Shorten nails with a nail clipper before shaping. Shape the nails with a quality-grade emery board or file. Gently file the nail on both sides, moving in one direction toward the center.

Step Three. Soak fingers in a nail bowl for several minutes and towel dry.

Step Four. Apply cuticle remover to the sides and base of nails and under nails. Gently push back cuticle with a manicure orange stick or cuticle shaper. Caution: be extremely careful when doing this procedure, even though I know it looks chic to be doing something else while giving yourself a manicure, like talking on the phone, as illustrated in magazines, etc. You can cause discomfort and sensitivity around the cuticle if you push too hard. Furthermore, if you are too rough, you can create dark areas around the cuticle. Be gentle! Always sterilize the cuticle area with alcohol or peroxide to prevent swelling and infection. Remove excess cuticle remover lotion from your nails by soaking them in peroxide.

Step Five. Clip excess cuticle and hangnails (if you must) with an implement trimmer or cuticle scissors. Apply an antibiotic ointment and leave on for a few minutes. Cleanse nails with warm soapy water. (Remove any excess polish with polish remover.)

Step Six. Smooth the nail surface and edges with a quality buffer. If you feel the nail mantle (the surface) getting warm and numb, you are removing too many layers of the nail. Be observant. If you take your time and concentrate, you can achieve nail salon perfection results. Remember to always buff in one direction.

Step Seven. Apply a clear base coat.

Step Eight. Apply two coats of nail polish: one broad stroke down the center and one on each side. Clean up any mess with a swab saturated in polish remover or plain ol' peroxide.

Step Nine. Apply quick-drying or speed-drying spray to the nails.

Step Ten. Pamper your lovely nails with a hand-softening cream with silky-smooth properties.

FYI

HAVE YOU GOT HANGNAILS?

If so, they are best left to a professional. But if you must treat them yourself, keep the nails clean and moist. Treat them to a little tea tree oil—great therapy!

FYI

Buffing can even out ridges on your nails and can aid in removing surface stains on your nails.

Different Special Effects for Nails

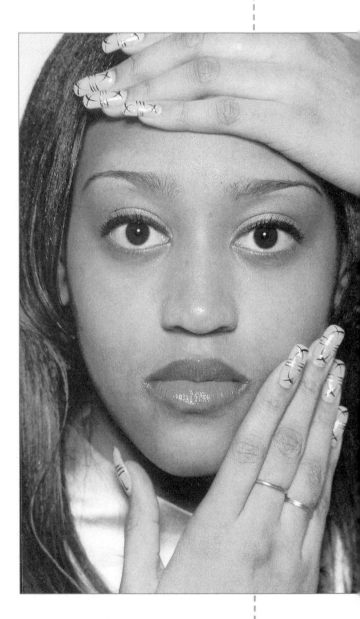

- Stencils come in a variety of cutout designs. After your nails are polished and dry, stick on your favorite shape, polish it in, and peel it off. *Voilà!*

- Nail art is good if you or someone you know is an artist. Dream up any design you want and paint it on dry polished nails in contrasting colors.

- Decals are little design shapes that stick to or adhere to your nail. Apply them on clear or dry polished nails and then paint over with a clear coat of polish or top coat.

- Jewels are little sparkly gems that you stick on for shimmery pizzazz. Apply them after you polish your nails and before they dry. Or to stick them on dry polish use the special nail adhesive that comes in the kit.

- The French manicure is very chic and classy. To achieve this look you first polish your nails in a neutral color like beige or light pink. Then you paint a coat of opaque white polish in a straight line across the tip of your nail. (Get help if you need it.) If you can't draw straight, try a French manicure kit with stick-on stencils.

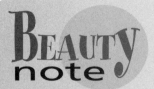

Weak, fragile, chipping, splitting, and peeling nails require regular conditioning treatment. Nail hardener, protein nail treatment, or liquid nail wrap are recommended.

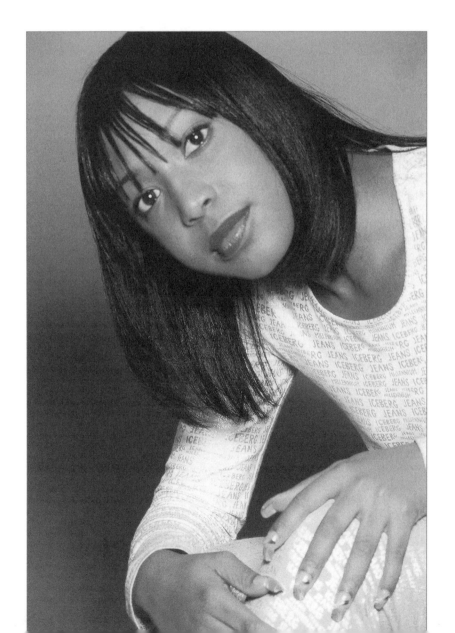

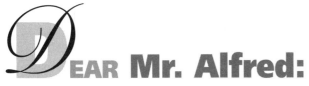

Dear Mr. Alfred:

My fingernails are always breaking. How can I make them stronger?

—JASMINE
Jacksonville, Florida, age 13

Dear Jasmine:

Always carry an emery board with you so you can get rid of snags right away. Keep your nails as short as you can stand until you treat them and make them stronger. The best way to do that is by massaging cuticle oil or a protein into them daily. Just use a clear, protective polish until you see improvement.

—MR. ALFRED

Pedicure Tools

- Nail Polish Remover
- Cotton Balls or Pads
- Emery Board or Emery File
- Nail Soak
- Cuticle Lotion Remover
- Manicure Orange Stick
- Toenail Clippers
- Pumice Stone or Foot Groomer
- Base Coat
- Nail Polish
- Quick-Drying or Speed-Drying Top Coat
- Creamy Foot-Moisturizing Conditioner

The Pedicure—Step up with Glorious Feet

To prepare for a pedicure, scrub your feet in the shower or bath, using a pumice stone or liquid rough-skin remover. This will gently smooth your feet.

Step One. Remove old nail polish.

Step Two. Trim the toenails with toenail clippers. With an emery board or emery file, round the corners of the toenails.

Steps Three to Ten. (Follow the same steps given in The Basic Manicure—Ten Steps to Fabulous Nails.)

GOT FOOT ODOR?

First of all, make sure to dry your feet thoroughly when you bathe or shower, and invest in a foot powder or spray. To keep the odor out of your shoes, try using some odor-absorbing insoles.

Special Stuff

When you do housework (especially when using water) always use rubber gloves.

Artificial nails are in fashion and come in great colors. Yes, they can be fun. So if you must, try them for special occasions.

Your own nails will be strong and long if you manicure them every week.

Make sure you eat a balanced diet. Calcium is good for your nails. Try milk, yogurt, cheese, and broccoli.

To soften your hands and feet, apply moisturizer and wear cotton socks or gloves to bed.

Creams with natural ingredients, such as keratin, protein, and vitamin E, are great for your hands and nails.

The 411 on Tattoos and Body Piercing

Tattooing: It's a Culture, Not Just a Trend

At one time, it was commonly thought that only people in motorcycle clubs and gangs wore tattoos. But rap, hip-hop, and R & B in our culture have opened up how a tattoo is viewed and valued by mainstream society. Social values are now more relaxed, and the tattoo has moved from being an "outsider" or "deviant" art form to being a more socially acceptable and admired art form. Tattoos have become more widely acceptable over the last ten years than in any other time in history. They have been popularized through their use in advertisements and by the BET and MTV crowd of the 1980s treading its way into the business offices of today's world. Tattoos can be seen as being status indicators, power symbols warn by warriors, criminal brands, deviant icons, and even "fad" body accessories. Tattoos can also be used as symbols for a unique group, such as gangs, fraternities, or certain cultures. The tattoo has represented many things to many people in many places.

Tattooing can often be very beautiful and can be your personal statement about who you are. Tattooing can make you stand out in a crowd, giving you a special dimension or individuality, or it can be an indication of your culture. In fact, the art of tattooing has evolved in many cultures worldwide, and thoughout history, it has been viewed in a variety of ways.

Henna has been used pretty expansively in the Middle East, where in places like Casablanca and Rabat women— older women wearing djellabas, young women in smart suits, high school students in jeans—can be seen on the bus or walking through town wearing henna tattoos.

Henna and how and when it is used varies greatly from culture to culture. In Morocco, for instance, henna tattoos are quite prevalent, and the patterns vary distinctly. For instance, in rural areas the designs are often cruder and thicker, with blunt designs and big geometric shapes, but in the cities, the designs are elaborate and very popular. Traditionally, a new bride, as well as all of her friends, has a big henna party where the bride gets most of the henna work and her friends get smaller designs on their hands or feet.

The art of tattooing has been transformed as a result of not only changes in social values but also those in power redefining mainstream values. Henna "tattoos" have traditionally been used by folkloric dancers, by Persian dancers, and by Native American tribal-style troupes. Henna designs are so diverse that they can appear in whole-arm designs worn by certain cultures or groups, and they are worn on the upper arm by fashion models! Hennaed "bracelets" have become a great accessory! But if you use henna as a fashion statement, you have one prime consideration—henna is *orange*. If you think orange designs would go well with your fashions, go for it!

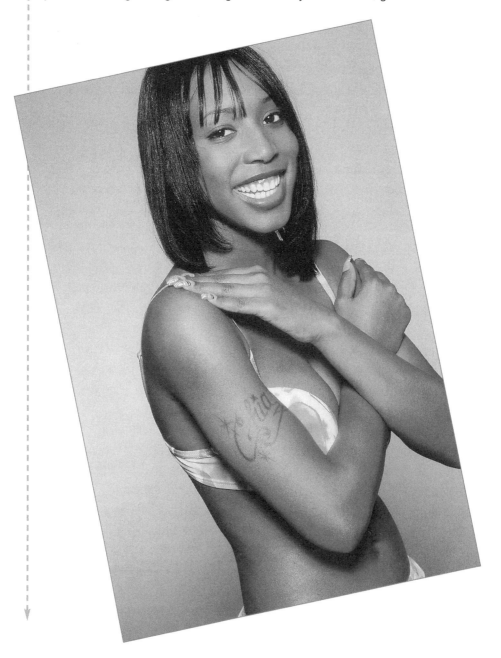

I asked a few teens what they thought about tattoos and body piercing and was pleasantly surprised by some of their comments.

I think that if you want a tattoo or piercing, just remember that it's always going to be there.

—JAMILAH

Mt. Vernon, New York, age 14

I have my name tattooed on my arm and I love it!

—LUCHIA

New York, New York, age 16

I don't like to mark my body. Some of my friends have them on their arms and legs—stupid stuff, like names and dogs. Some boys like them on girls, but I think most of them think a girl is wild if she wears them. Anything you do like that could affect your professional life as an adult.

—TYEKA

Boston, Massachusetts, age 16

According to Dr. Susan Taylor, "Body tattooing, again, can be very painful. It is permanent. Lasers can remove them, although quite often it just lightens the tattoo. It can be surgically removed, but then you're left with a scar. I don't think it is safe to tattoo the breast or the nipple area. And I'm absolutely horrified by tattooing the vaginal area—I think one should avoid that."

Natural Henna Tattoos

Want a safe and temporary way to tattoo? Can you or your friends draw or sketch fun designs? Try something different with a group of your friends or sisters—have a henna party (with permission, of course)! It's fun, interesting, cultural, safe—and the designs look great! And very few people are allergic to traditional henna. If you have a henna tattoo, be proud. Enjoy it.

1. Buy your henna. First, you'll need some henna powder. Make sure your henna is of good quality. Buy it in little boxes at Indian grocery stores. The bulk henna sold at health food stores just doesn't give as good a color in comparison. If your henna powder has twigs and things in it, be sure to sift it before you mix it! (If you sift out the clumpy bits of sticks, then you can get much finer designs than if you use it straight out of the box.)

2. Mix your henna. Take about a tablespoon full of henna powder and put it in a plastic bowl. Empty yogurt containers work well.

    You will need boiling water, preferably bottled or distilled, though the tap water isn't a problem. Now—here comes the big secret! Boil dried limes in water until the water turns red. (This really happens!) It seems to work much better if you first cut up your limes and dry them in slices, rather than using them whole. Dry three to six limes at a time. (You may lose a few pieces to mold.) Use all the limes you have on hand to make the "broth" and add the boiling water to make a paste. Let it cool down or "set" for about twenty minutes before applying, so it can do its thing.

Alternative

Fresh limes don't work the same way! If you're out of dried limes, then just add either lemon or lime juice to the henna (at least two tablespoons). Take a fresh lemon and squeeze it. Pour the juice through a sieve to remove any pulp, as this will clog your applicator. Add a couple of teaspoons of the strained lemon juice to the henna powder. Mix together (use a plastic spoon) and add more lemon juice until you get a thick paste. (Over time you'll get used to judging how much liquid to pour in.) To store it, just cover the bowl with plastic wrap.

Want More Color?

If you want to add extra ingredients to darken the final color, try a few drops of clove oil or about half a teaspoon of clove (make sure that you are not allergic). Mix thoroughly.

The Application Process

Your hands (or feet, or whatever) must be clean and free from moisturizers, lotions, grease, oils, or other goop, which would all prevent your henna from being absorbed!

Henna painting can be done with toothpicks, orange sticks, syringes, and tubes—but the make-it-yourself funnel has been claimed as the best and easiest method (pastry tubes don't work as well because it's hard to get the henna out past the tip). This is a great trick. Take a heavy-duty plastic bag (like you get at women's clothing stores) and cut a piece out, twist it into a funnel, and pin it together. Fill it with henna, and you have the neatest, most precise tool! You could also try a heavy plastic shopping bag cut into squares and rolled into tubes, secured with either tape or a straight pin, or even a Ziploc bag. Orange sticks are invaluable for touching up designs or straightening lines. (Toothpicks are usable but are a bit too small.) Once your design is applied, it will start to dry and crack. Fill in the cracks with a thinned-down henna paste until you have a more-or-less even coat of drying green goo. Then you can moisten the henna with a mixture of water and lemon or lime juice. (Try adding sugar. In Morocco, they use sugar water for moistening.) Moisten the henna at least three times, letting it dry most of the way in between.

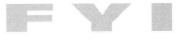

The Earth Henna Kit from Lakaye Mehndi is the easiest kit for applications that we know of. This kit comes complete with henna powder, easy-to-use premeasured henna solution, which increases the shelf life of the henna for up to one month, eucalyptus oil, reusable applicator bottle with metal tip, stencils, cotton tips, and toothpicks.

Your henna tattoo will set better if it dries with heat. So, if you can, stick your hands in the sun, or dry them around a candle flame (this is hard!), or use a hair dryer.

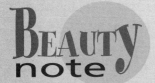

The length of time it takes the henna to dry depends on how thick the paste is. Be careful with a thick, large design, keeping an eye on it until it really starts to dry, or you could mess up the design. The longer you leave the paste on, the longer it will last and the darker the color will be. For some hand designs, you can wrap it with gauze and sleep with it on!

For best results, leave your henna on for at least an hour, or for as long as you can stand it. When you finally remove it, make sure to scrape it off. Don't just wash it off. If your first attempt didn't come out very dark, you can apply henna again, right over the first design. It is very easy to apply this way— having the design to follow makes it *a lot* easier! (Keep toothpicks and orange sticks on hand to clean up the lines of your design. Henna *will* dye your nails permanently! It takes a long time to grow out! Be warned! If you don't want orange fingernails for the next four months, put some nail polish on before you start the process. At any rate, try not to get the mixture on your nails.

WHICH TYPE OF HENNA IS BEST?

Stick with natural, or traditional henna. It is a natural plant dye that colors the skin orange/brown. It is safe because the dye in henna penetrates only as far as the outer dead skin cells—the epidermis. You can tell if your henna artist is using safe henna because the stain will be orange/brown and the paste will not be jet black. The artist should be able to tell you what ingredients have been used.

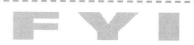
"Black Henna" Temporary Tattoos May Be Hazardous to Your Health

Clients who don't know the dangers connected with black henna sometimes prefer the black look, as it looks similar to a permanent tattoo.

Black henna is natural henna mixed with a black dye, which gives a long-lasting jet black color. Natural henna can go almost black on the palm in high heat, and other safer ingredients exist. But none rapidly gives the jet black look that black henna can. This is because the dye used in black henna is PPD (phenylenediamine), a black chemical dye often used as hair dye. Unfortunately, when applied to the skin it can cause an allergic reaction in some people—anything from a slight rash to blisters, oozing sores, intense itching, and long-term scarring. Before you get any tattoo, always ask the artist what ingredients are being used. If they can't tell you, walk away. If they can, judge what they say for yourself. If the paste is jet black, walk away. If the stain is jet black, took less than two hours to go black, and lasts for ten days or more, it's PPD.

Temporary Tattoos

Make a statement with a temporary tattoo. They are quick and easy to apply, and you can change designs whenever you want a new look. (Check ingredients to make sure there are no dye products that you might be allergic to.) Some of the designs you can get include: armbands, hearts and love, barbed-wire henna, birds, butterflies, dragon-flies, cartoon characters, crosses, stars, moons, dragons, snakes, fantasy suns, super-heros, flowers, tribal designs, and wild beasts.

Keep in mind the varied choices available today—older designs, work done by a loved one, even abstract pieces. If you take a look inside your local tattoo studio, you will see the difference between what it "was" yesterday, and what it "is" today. Many of the artists have split into specialties and are doing what they say is their best work. Don't be swayed by any voice except your own. If you choose to tattoo, take your time to select the art that represents you, but always remember, if you choose a permanent tattoo, it may be a lifelong statement.

Body Piercing

Just like tattooing, body piercing has cultural roots. Body modification, enhancement, and adornment have all been a part of human culture throughout history. It's an art form that has been used by hundreds of tribes throughout the world for centuries—as both status symbols as well as an art form. Naval piercing was a symbol of royalty among ancient Egyptians, and Amazonian tribal hunters and gatherers wore bull rings to look more fearsome so they could intimidate their prey. A lot of girls get body piercings because their friends do. Again, consider your uniqueness when choosing this accessory, and use good judgment to decide when and where to pierce.

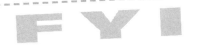

Hygiene and safety are the chief concerns of critics of body piercing. The increased popularity of piercing has led to several cases of infection and injuries.

Dr. Taylor states, "Body piercing is a fad. People can develop keloids from it. You must always consider that. If you wear earrings that are too heavy, the ears can become torn, but they can be repaired safely. Be careful with tongue piercing—you don't want to choke on the earring."

QUIZ   THOSE EXTRA ACCENTS THAT DEFINE YOU

1
Q. Which is stronger, perfume or cologne?
A. Perfume is the strongest of all types of fragrance.

2
Q. Should you share your fragrances with your friends?
A. No, because fragrances react differently on everyone and might not smell good on someone else.

3
Q. What is the best type of water to bathe in?
A. Use warm, tepid water—never hot.

4
Q. What do you do with a buffer?
A. Smooth the nail surfaces and edges.

5
Q. How can you tell if your henna artist is using safe henna?
A. Because the stain will be orange/brown and the paste will not be jet black.

6
Q. What can happen if you wear earrings that are too heavy?
A. Your ear can tear.

CHAPTER 5

Chic Hairstyles and Care for Your Hair

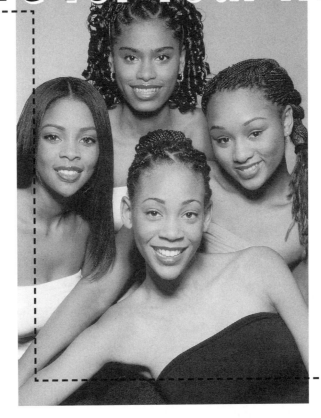

THERE'S SO MUCH TO KNOW about your hair. During your lifetime, you will probably wear a number of different styles and lengths, and perhaps even a number of different colors.

How Should I Wear My Hair?

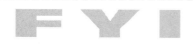

MOISTURE MEANS A LOT

Just as you take care of your skin by using daily moisturizers, you should satisfy your hair's craving for moisture. There are a host of products available that penetrate the cells of your hair to keep it soft, glowing, and healthy.

You are so lucky! Depending on how you have it styled, your hair can be straight, curly, waved, naturally kinky, or anything in between. You can wear a diverse range of looks, from short and sassy, long and layered, flowing curls, classic bobs, elegant up-dos, tantalizing twists, smoothed back, beautiful braids, ponytails, or loose.

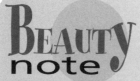 Avocado can be more than a meal! Before you shampoo, precondition your hair with avocado. Use half of a ripe avocado mashed or blended well. For great results, massage it into your hair and leave it on for fifteen minutes.

Black teens don't all have the same kind of hair—there are eighteen different follicle types, which come in coarse, medium, and fine textures. For a great look, the challenge is to find your own best style.

Look for a style that complements your face shape. See pages 88–90 to help you determine your face shape. Pull your hair back and check it out.

- *Oblong.* Your chin is long and your forehead is high. Choose soft, rounded styles, which do not lengthen the face. One such method is to have a feathery bang. Hair looks best at jaw length, full and off the face. If you decide to wear your hair long, avoid a straight look.

- *Oval.* This face is balanced, with chin and forehead about the same size. Lucky you! Oval is considered to be the perfect model shape. Just about any hairstyle will fit the oval face's features. Choose a style that best suits your hair texture and type. Your choices can include bobs, braids, weaves, curls, waves, or straight looks.

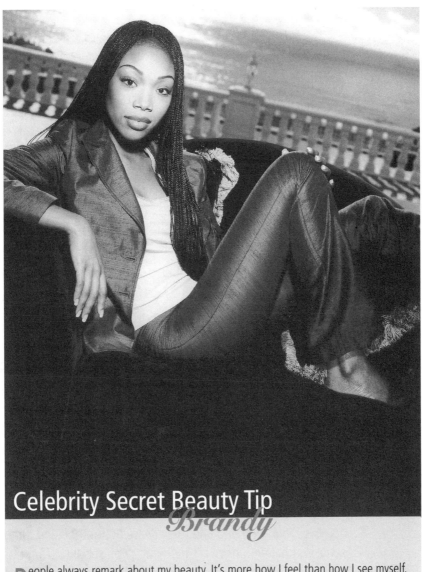

Celebrity Secret Beauty Tip
Brandy

People always remark about my beauty. It's more how I feel than how I see myself, though. I surround myself with positive people, stay low, keep moving, and believe in God.

Round. This face shape is rather full, especially at the cheeks. You should build as much height as possible with your hair—this will give the look of length to your face. Avoid framing your face with too much hair, particularly with thickness at ear length. Clean, straight lines will contour and slenderize your face. An excellent choice for a round face is a bob cut.

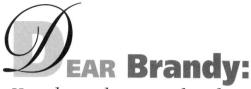

DEAR Brandy:

How do you keep your braids so beautiful?

—JASMINE
Jacksonville, Florida, age 13

Dear Jasmine:

I keep my scalp well conditioned, and I have a personal hair and braid stylist who even travels with me when I'm on tour.

—BRANDY

TEEN TIP

My bangs were causing me to break out on my forehead. So at night I tie a small cotton scarf under my bangs, around my head, and then of course tie on a silk scarf to keep my hair from tangling and breaking.

—ALLYSON
Dayton, Ohio, age 14

STYLING SUGGESTION

Quick and easy! Hairpieces can be very appealing and add versatility to your look. Try a chignon, upsweep, topknot, or ponytail, for example, for a collection of effects from casual to sophisticated.

- *Square.* Your forehead and jawline are both broad and almost the same width. If you have a square face, you should soften the lines, both on your forehead and chin, by having your hair fall gently to those areas. Asymmetrical styles, layered cuts, or soft waves work well to flatter the squareness of your face.

- *Heart.* Your forehead and cheeks will be the widest parts of the face, which gets narrowest at the chin. For a heart-shaped face, you may opt to wear a flip with a soft-cropped bang. This will give an illusion of fullness in your cheek area.

- *Pear.* Your jawline and cheeks are fuller than your forehead. To add balance to a pear-shaped face, wear your hair short and full. Keep it cropped at ear length for best results.

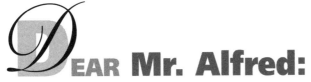

DEAR Mr. Alfred:

I just moved to a new community and I'm so upset because my hairstylist is so far away. What's the best way to find a new stylist without getting burned?

—ALICIA
St. Louis, Missouri, age 16

Dear Alicia:

Ask around in school or at church to find out who the best hairstylists are in your neighborhood. If you see someone wearing a look that you like, ask them who they used.

—MR. ALFRED

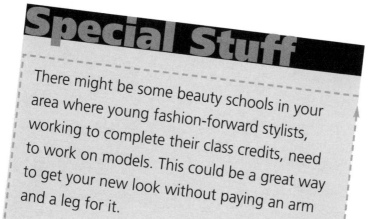

Special Stuff

There might be some beauty schools in your area where young fashion-forward stylists, working to complete their class credits, need to work on models. This could be a great way to get your new look without paying an arm and a leg for it.

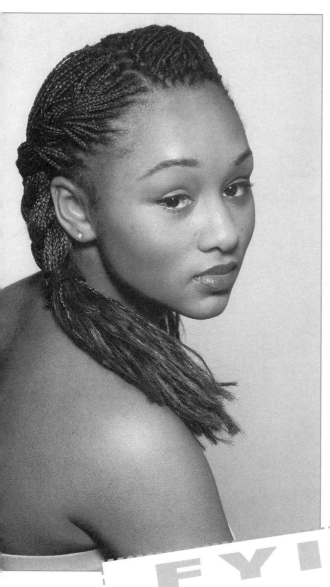

Hair Weaves, Braids, and Extensions

These alternatives include getting a full weave, braids, or just a few tracks to add fullness and length to your own hair. For those of you who have not tried either technique, here are a few details:

Full Weaves

A full weave is done on your entire head in either of two methods. All your natural hair can be cornrowed in a flat braid around your entire head. Wefts of hair are then sewn onto the tracks in the best direction to fall into the shape that you desire. (You can choose any texture, quality, color, or length of hair—preferably human hair.) Once all of the hair is sewn on, it will be cut and styled as you wish.

FYI

Instead of having wefts of hair sewn on, you can have them glued to your scalp with a special glue. (This is not a preferred technique. It might cause damage if they are not removed properly.)

Braids

There are so many styles to choose from! Have fun with this in a style that's long or short, braids (or twists) that are thick or thin, loose and long, or cornrowed and contoured. Synthetic hair is best for braided styles—again, choose your favorite color.

Interlocking

This is also a form of braiding, but it resembles a weave. Your natural hair is braided individually, with hair extensions mixed in, then locked or knotted close to the scalp. This looks very natural—the hair remains loose and full, creating a weave look. (Always use human hair for this look.)

Natural Styles

If your hair is naturally curly, why straighten it with chemicals? Wear it with pride. And those short Afros are quite chic too. But growing in trendiness is the loc. Locs are a fashion statement unto themselves. Whether it's for spiritual reasons, as an affirmation of power, or just plain fashion sense, if you opt for locs, you're a brave little sister. The process of loc'ing the hair takes from about three to six months. During this time, your hair will go through several stages, some very difficult to manage. For best results, I strongly recommend getting it started professionally by a loctician. Every few months thereafter, treat yourself to a professional grooming, to make sure that your hair is cleaned thoroughly and properly conditioned. Between appointments, however, be sure to clean and moisturize your hair and scalp regularly.

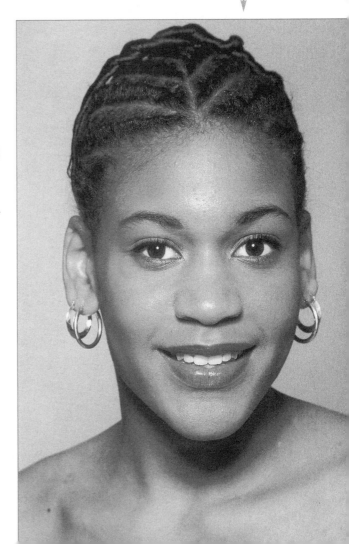

Straightened Hair

By taking the curl or the kink out of your hair, it will become straightened, which will greatly expand your styling choices. Before chemical relaxers were developed, everyone straightened (pressed) their hair with a pressing comb and then curled it with curling irons or set it on rollers. But, of course, this had to be done every time your hair was shampooed. I do believe that before chemical relaxers were developed, hair was much healthier and maintained its thickness much longer. Today, chemical straightening is quicker and lasts much longer, but your poor hair suffers. Overprocessing and under-conditioning are the two biggest culprits.

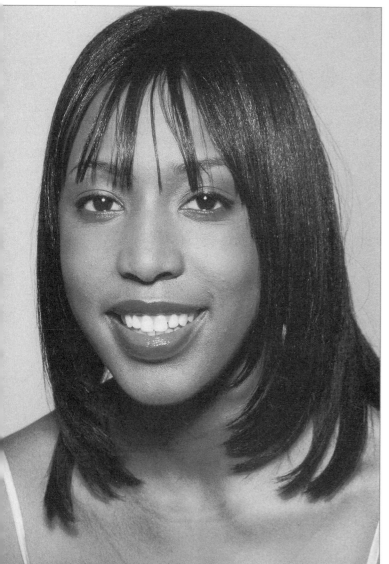

Of course, chemical relaxers are the most popular method of hair straightening and the most important step toward getting the style of your choice, but I caution you to use care. Know your stylist, or if you do it yourself, read and follow the directions completely. Once you have relaxed your hair, you can usually get the cut or shape that you want. Enjoy!

Now Let's Do Color!

When I was beauty editor at *Ebony* and *Essence* magazines, people always asked me: "What are the newest trends in hair-grooming products for teens of color?" The answer is obvious: the African American teenager wants more color in her life. She wants to enhance and highlight her otherwise very dark hair. What was perceived as a trend then is now an avalanche.

African American teenagers at major black college campuses established the new style with colored natural, chemically treated plaits, twists, braids, different colored hair wigs, and extensions. New York, Chicago, Los Angeles, and Atlanta have exploded with teenagers flaunting complementary blonde, red, brunette, brown, and of course black. My favorite new hair colorings are the fabulous berry shades and hues of highlights that range from strawberry blondes to plum henna tones on natural, untreated hair. The rich deep beiges, golden bronzes, and high-sheen browns enlivened with streaks of champagne blonde, apricot, cinnamon, and chestnut are just fantastic! I'm convinced that some "blondes do have more fun" too! Variety is now available and good choices can be made, though the look may be redefined and updated for the future. But hair coloring as a fashion statement is definitely here to stay!

Like your skin undertone, your hair has a tone that ranges from yellow-gold or yellow-red to red, and dark red or red-brown to brown-black. Your eye color and natural hair color are your best guides in choosing the correct hair color. My color chart, designed especially for you, can help you make the best choices. I strongly suggest that you consult a haircolor specialist at your beauty salon before you color your hair. If you do consider coloring your hair at home, I urge you to read the manufacturer's guide for better hair coloring; and by all means, don't mix color with any other hair chemicals.

The best guide to choosing a hair color is a strand test, which you can do yourself. Test a strand or section of your hair to see how the new color will relate to your eyes and skin. Also, determine how the change will make you feel—before going all the way. Take a strand from underneath your outer layer of hair so it won't show if you should decide not to proceed. The strand test can be done under the supervision of your hair colorist or at home with an over-the-counter color product.

Whichever coloring process you choose—home or salon—always make sure you or your stylist completely understands the instructions. Here are the basic types of hair color:

Henna

This is one of the most popular natural plant dyes with American black teenagers who wear their hair short and tapered close to the sides and nape of the neck. Henna comes in different colors and produces various effects. It can give the hair rich, deep, lustrous appeal, or give natural hair a healthy, bright glow. Henna is free of ammonia and peroxide.

Vegetable Dye

Like henna, vegetable dyes are free from ammonia and peroxide. A variety of vegetable juices and fruits, particularly berries, stain the surface of the hair shaft and penetrate it to produce a bright or rich, deep-textured appearance of the hair. This sure beats boiling Kool-Aid, or cranberry and lemon juices, individually or as a cocktail colorant, which often produced those awful, flat colors that would take a week or two to shampoo out.

Temporary Color

These are shampoo-in, styling gels, tints, creams, soufflés, mousses, and spray formulas that are nonalkaline and free from ammonia and peroxide, and they work gently with

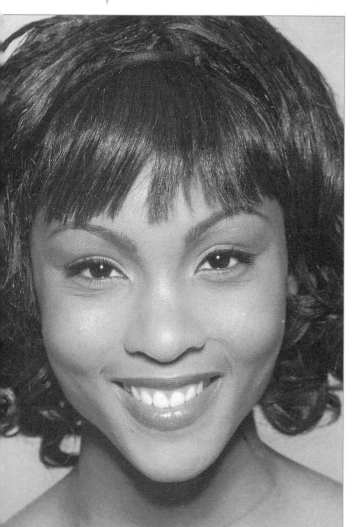

the natural chemistry of your hair. Temporary colors coat the surface of the hair shaft and will wash out literally with the next shampoo. They are excellent for permed or relaxed hair. Always consult the manufacturer's product claims in the brand's insert for guidance.

Semipermanent Color

These are designed to coat, surround, and cling to the outer cuticle shaft of the hair. Semipermanent colors start to rinse off after four to six washings. Some semipermanent color products contain peroxide (a hair-lightening ingredient on some hair types). Always do a strand test, particularly if your hair has been chemically treated.

Permanent Color

This is full strength and long lasting. Teenage girls should be extremely careful with this one. Permanent color changes the character pigment balance and natural hair color and is best applied in a salon by a professional hair colorist, particularly if you are insecure about your first color change. Permanent hair color products last longer than any other hair coloring. Special care for permed and relaxed hair is advised; and NEVER, NEVER use permanent hair coloring the same day that you perm or relax your hair!

There are other natural and synthetic ways to change your hair color or give your hair highlights, including comb-in hair color and colored sprays for spot application of hair color.

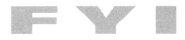

Temporary applications of pomade are not recommended for most African American hair textures. Removing the stuff from your hair is just an awful, messy experience.

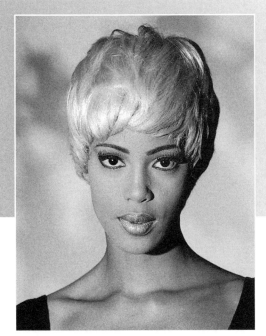

Style Suggestion

Before you drastically change your hair with a new cut or color, I recommend that you go to a store and try on some wigs so that you can see how you will look in the style that you are considering.

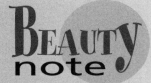

Highlights and streaks are great ways to add color to your hair without getting an allover change. And they've even got great pin-in hairpieces for that extra pizzazz.

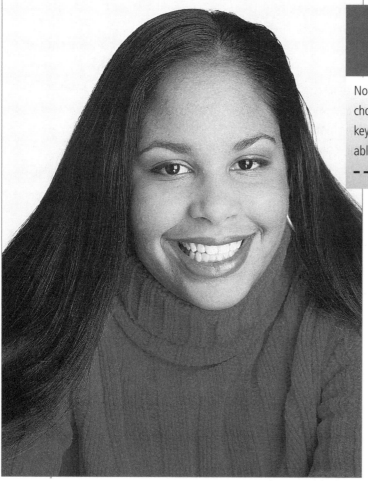

CONDITION, CONDITION, CONDITION!

No matter which hairstyle you choose, conditioning your hair is key to maintaining your fashionable well-groomed look

----

For those of you who choose to color your hair, there are some great shampoos especially formulated for your hair. Used according to the instructions, they will maintain the health, softness, and vibrancy of your hair. If you follow up your shampoo with complementary conditioners (always use the same brands), you should be able to

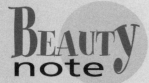

BEAUTY note

Be true to yourself! No matter what look you get, it's got to feel good to you. A lot of my teenage customers ask for braids or weaves. I always advise them not to get a style just because their friend is wearing it or because they saw it on a celebrity. Know your face shape and your lifestyle and understand the maintenance requirements. If it fits you all-round, by all means, do it!

—Grace Monica, Grace Monica Salon, Brooklyn, New York

keep your hair from becoming dry, brittle, and dull. Ask your stylist for the best product lines for your special type of hair.

Here's some stuff to help you take care of your hair, keep it fresh and chic, and add a little glam.

Best Tools for Styling Your Hair

- Natural boar bristle brushes are good if you wear your hair natural or if it has been chemically treated. They won't snag and break your hair like brushes with nylon or synthetic bristles.
- Rubber bristle brushes with large round tips are good if your hair is weaved.
- Combs are for detangling or smoothing your hair. Wide-tooth rubber combs are unquestionably the preferred tool for you. They also work well for combing conditioner through your hair while you are in the shower.
- Picks are good for natural hair. If you are wearing an Afro, or if your hair is very curly, this is a must-have.

Blow Dryers

Whatever fits your hands best can work. Be sure that you don't have the heat too high if your hair is chemically processed.

Curlers and Straightening Combs

- If you want to change your straight hairstyle pronto, curl the ends with an electric curling iron. Watch that heat, though.
- Rollers that use steam are great for keeping the moisture in your hair, if you've got the time to sit for a while.
- Plastic or metal rollers work well for a wet set, but always use end papers first, to keep ends from catching and breaking.
- Straightening combs are available in electric or stove-top styles. In both cases watch the temperature—these will burn your hair if they get too hot.

Those Little Extras

- Barrettes
- Bobby Pins
- Hair Pins
- Headbands
- Coated Rubber Hair Bands
- Hair Clips
- Clip-on Hairpieces
- Sparkles

Hair-Care Supplies

- Shampoo (alternate between those with and without built-in conditioners)

- Instant conditioners for regular weekly or biweekly shampoos

- Deep-penetrating conditioners with protein or other natural ingredients for one or two treatments per month.

- Hair moisturizer or oil for daily scalp treatment and hair grooming

- Hair gel for quick slick looks

- Hair mousse for fun full styles

- Hair spray to keep it all together

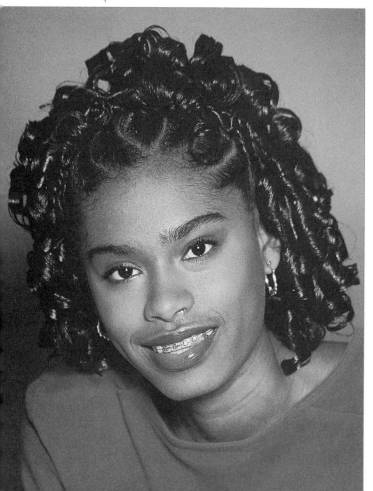

Hair's the Facts

- Your hair grows about half an inch a month.

- Don't worry if you see a little shedding when you comb. Hair sheds too, just like skin does when you bathe.

- Regular trims are okay and they keep the splits away!

Speaking of Hair!

If you are experiencing excess facial hair, don't panic. Some females just have more facial hair than others, and most often, it's hereditary. You might have sideburns, hairs on the temples, cheeks, upper lips, under the lower lip, or chin hairs. I am not against your shaving your legs, but I am definitely against your shaving the facial area. Often hairs in the facial area will grow back more coarse and this stubble will create more of a problem for continued removal. And, when you shave, there is a major concern that scarring could be permanent. Your mother probably has firsthand knowledge about facial hair removal, or ask your pharmacist about gentle-strength over-the-counter hair removers, formulated specifically for teenagers. You may also wish to explore professional services. Find out which ones are teenage friendly and reserve an evening or weekend day to visit with them. Here are some types of professional services.

Hair Wax Removal

Hair wax removal is my first recommendation. Wax is a natural ingredient that is not loaded with harsh, irritating chemicals. When you remove hairs by waxing, the skin is left smooth, hairs grow back at a slower rate, and when they reappear, they feel soft, not stubbly and coarse. This temporary process leaves the skin smooth and is an efficient way to remove hair from large and small areas. I suggest that you first experience waxing in a professional environment, and then, if you prefer, try an over-the-counter product at home. There are hot and cold methods, which work equally well. More and more nail salons are offering hair-waxing services. Most spas and beauty salons that do hair removal will recommend consultation with an aesthetician or licensed cosmetologist, who specializes in various methods of hair removal.

Tweezing

With tweezing, you will remove each hair individually. This is a temporary method, as hair will grow back and you'll have to tweeze on a regular basis. Scarring could occur, so you must be extremely careful, and if you have a tendency to scar, this method should be avoided.

Electrolysis

Another method of hair removal is electrolysis. African American teenagers must be extremely cautious with this method, as you can get scars from overstimulating the pore opening. This permanent procedure is done by electric currents, so you risk the possibility of electric shock and infection from an incompetent aesthetician. Above all, electrolysis can become quite expensive. If you do consider this method, be sure to get a second opinion and some testimonies and/or view photos of past customers.

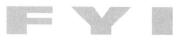

Your hair is in its weakest state when it's wet. So don't pull it. Always condition it before you comb so that you don't get tangles and break it. Also, keep your combs and brushes clean. Don't share your tools. Bacteria, lice, and dandruff can spread.

QUIZ   HAIRSTYLES AND HAIR CARE

1
Q. What face shape do they call the perfect model look?
A. Oval.

2
Q. What type of hair color lasts the longest?
A. Permanent.

3
Q. What type of hair is recommended for braids?
A. Synthetic hair.

4
Q. When should you do a strand test?
A. Before you color your hair.

5
Q. What kind of rollers keep the moisture in your hair?
A. Rollers that use steam are best.

6
Q. What is the best type of comb to use for your hair type?
A. A wide-tooth rubber comb.

CHAPTER 6

Food, Fashion, and Fitness for a Better You

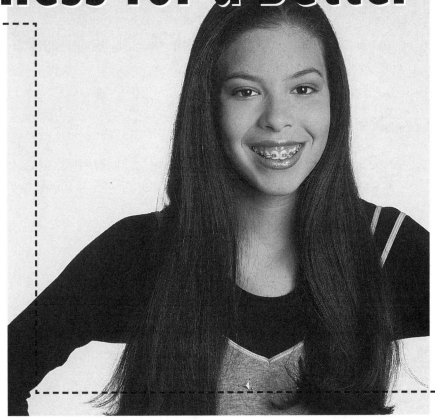

M ANY FACETS ARE INVOLVED in making you as beautiful as you are. We've talked extensively about your skin, makeup, colors, and hair. Let's spend a little time now on your physical self—being fit and fabulous!

Fast Break

The most important meal—hands down—is BREAKFAST! After resting (or fasting) all night, your body now needs to be refueled and reenergized to meet the needs of a new day. Don't make a "fast break" for the door without stopping for refueling; take time to "break the fast."

A Few Quick Healthy Choices

- Bowl of hot or cold cereal with milk (try soy milk, you might like it), topped with fruit.

- Bagel with melted cheese or peanut butter, and fruit or juice.

- Yogurt parfait (alternate layers of plain/lemon/vanilla yogurt) with fruit and topped with cereal (such as granola).

Snacks

Snacks can be a quick-and-easy way to refuel your body. Just remember that frequent snacking also means you are increasing your caloric intake. Snacks should not replace meals.

Quick Pick-Me-Up Snacks

- Cottage cheese/fruit

- Yogurt parfait

- Flavored rice cakes or corn cakes, with peanut butter

- Apple slices and cheese slices

- Homemade trail mix. Add or delete the foods of your choice:

    $1/4$ cup low-sugar cereal (add Kix or Cheerios)

    $1/4$ cup nuts/seeds (add sunflower seeds, peanuts, or almonds)

    $1/4$ cup dried fruit and raisins? Maybe!

    $1/4$ cup pretzels

Got a Sweet Tooth?

Desserts are a wonderful part of your diet, and you need not deny yourself. Just don't overdo them. When you have the great sweet urge, consider one of the following:

Sweet Treats

- Angel food cake with fresh strawberries
- Small bowl of ice cream topped with fresh fruit
- Muffins, banana bread, cranberry bread, zucchini bread
- Fruit salad
- Half a grapefruit with a sprinkling of sugar
- Homemade milkshake with fruit (combine skim milk with ice milk or low-fat ice cream)

Watch Out for Weight Gain

- Limit sweets and fatty foods.
- Choose snacks wisely. Avoid mountains of empty-calorie foods such as chips, cookies, candy bars. They are full of calories but low in nutrients. The closer a food is to its natural state, the healthier it usually is for you.
- If your favorite food is also high in fat, don't deny yourself, just don't eat it daily.
- Read nutrition labels carefully. The higher the number of ingredients, the more processed (refined) it may be. This removes many vitamins that may not be added back. The less processed the food, usually the lower it is in fat.
- Watch out for "sneaky calories." These are sneaky because they taste good and are high in calories but provide little or no nutrition. For that reason, salad dressings, mayonnaise, butter, sugar, and oils should all be used sparingly.
- Beware of "liquid calories." Drinks like soda pop and caffe lattes are full of sneaky calories. *Reading labels is a must!* If a label uses *punch, cocktail,* or *-ade,* then sugar has been added.

Water

According to Sharmyn Phipps, a dietician and nutritional adviser, your body has a strong need for water.

How Your Body Uses Water

- Mode of transportation for nutrients to enter the cells.
- Mode of transportation for waste products to exit the body.
- Shock absorber, joint lubricant, and much more!

Is it hard to imagine drinking six to eight glasses a day? Try bottled flavored waters. These are cheaper per bottle than soda pop when bought by the case. Or add a slice of lemon or lime to your water. Or make your own flavored water by mixing carbonated water with a little 100 percent fruit juice. Fluids from other drinks such as juice and tea do count. Just remember to choose caffeine-free drinks, because caffeine does act as a diuretic in the body, flushing the needed water right out, thus increasing your need for water even more!

Try Vegetarian Nutrition

Reed Mangels, Ph.D., R.D., nutrition adviser for the Vegetarian Resource Group, states, "More teenagers are choosing not to eat meat, poultry, or fish." The following information was taken from his newsletter for teenagers. (For more information, write to The Vegetarian Resource Group, Box 1463, Baltimore, MD 21203, and check out their Web site: www.vrg.org.)

Vegetarians do not eat meat, fish, and poultry. Most vegetarians abstain from eating or using all animal products, including milk, cheese, other dairy items, and eggs. Among the many reasons for being a vegetarian are your health, ecological and religious concerns, dislike for meat, compassion for animals, belief in nonviolence, and economics.

The American Dietetic Association has affirmed that a vegetarian diet can supply all known nutrient needs.

The key to a healthy vegetarian diet, as with any other diet, is to eat a wide variety of foods, including fruits, vegetables, plenty of leafy greens, whole grain products, nuts, seeds, and legumes.

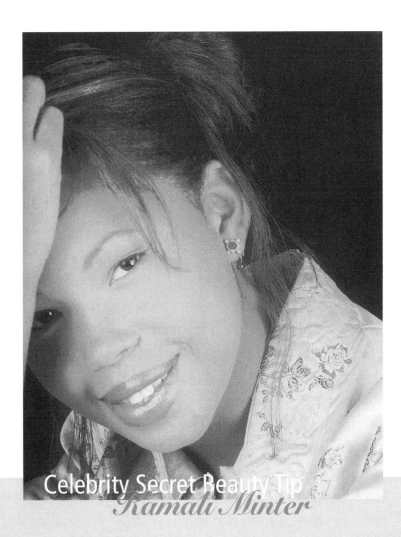

Celebrity Secret Beauty Tip
Kamali Minter

Many entertainers have opted to go vegetarian because of the obvious benefits of nourishing themselves with foods that won't weigh them down. Among those who indulge in this healthy lifestyle are Janet Jackson, Prince, and budding starlet Kamali Minter. As an actress, Kamali has been featured in numerous television programs, such as *Law and Order* and Hallmark Hall of Fame's "The Runaway," with Debbi Morgan and Maya Angelou.

Kamali states, "Looking your best is a process that begins on the inside. It is a harmonious balance between your mind, body, and spirit, which must be in good condition, in order for you to radiate the beauty that attracts attention. I know that no matter how sharp my clothes are or how well I hook up my hair and makeup, if I forget the hundreds of sit-ups and my five-day fast, then I am not at peace with myself. I may look good, but I will not be happy. Take time out of your day for yourself, even if it's just fifteen minutes when you first wake up, and absorb all the things you have to be thankful for. I like to meditate or write to center myself and rediscover my purpose.

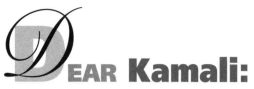

DEAR Kamali:

I'm thinking of making a lifestyle change beginning with a better diet. My mother doesn't support my desire to become a vegetarian and insists that I don't know what I'm doing or why I'm doing it. What should I tell her?

—JASMINE
Columbus, Georgia, age 16

Dear Jasmine:

I have been a vegetarian my whole life and have found that diet in combination with exercise and spiritual enrichment have been essential to looking and feeling good.

There are all kinds of ways that people go vegetarian and all kinds of reasons they do it. The basic definition is one who doesn't eat meat, but they might eat fish or eggs. On the other hand, I have been a vegan (a strict vegetarian who eats only vegetables) all my life, having grown up in a vegetarian household. Even though I was raised in a vegan household, at some point I made the decision to continue eating this way myself—it helps keep me healthy, energized, and slender. Let your mother know that your decision has been well thought out.

—KAMALI MINTER,
actress, director, graduate of NYU's Tisch School of the Arts

For a Healthy Vegetarian Diet, Variety Is the Key

The most important concern for teenage vegetarians is the nutritional adequacy of their food choices. A vegetarian diet can be enjoyed by people of all ages, but the key to a healthy vegetarian diet is variety. Just as your parents would be concerned if you ate only hamburgers, they would also worry if you only eat potato chips and salad. A healthy and varied vegetarian diet includes fruits, vegetables, plenty of leafy greens, whole grain products, nuts, seeds, and legumes. Some vegetarians also choose to eat dairy products and/or eggs.

Teenage vegetarians have nutritional needs that are the same as any other teenager. The years between thirteen and nineteen are times of especially rapid growth and change, so nutritional needs are high during these years. The nutrients that you will probably be asked about the most are protein, calcium, iron, and vitamin B_{12}.

What about Protein?

North American vegetarian teens eating varied diets rarely have any difficulty getting enough protein, as long as their diet contains enough energy (calories) to support growth. Cow's milk and low-fat cheese are protein sources; however, beans, breads, cereals, nuts, peanut butter, tofu, and soy milk are also some foods that are especially good sources of protein. Only fruits, fats, sugars, and alcohol do not provide much

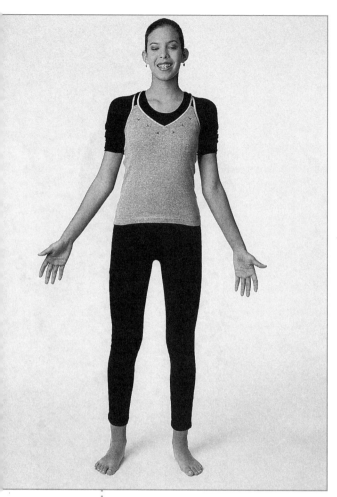

protein, so a diet based only on these foods would probably be too low in protein. It is not necessary to plan combinations of foods to obtain enough protein or amino acids, which are components of protein. A mixture of plant proteins eaten throughout the day will provide enough essential amino acids.

Other Important Nutrients

Especially during adolescence, calcium is needed to build bones. Bone density is determined in adolescence and young adulthood, so it is important to include three or more good sources of calcium in your diet every day. Cow's milk and dairy products do contain calcium. However, there are other good sources of calcium sulfate: tahini (sesame butter); green leafy vegetables, including collard greens, mustard greens, and kale; calcium-fortified soy milk and orange juice.

Iron requirements of teenagers are relatively high. By eating a vegetarian diet, a vegetarian can meet iron needs while avoiding the excess fat and cholesterol found in red meats such as beef or pork. To increase the amount of iron absorbed from a meal, eat a food containing vitamin C as part of the meal. Citrus fruits and juices (for example, orange juice), tomatoes, and broccoli are all good sources of vitamin C. Foods that are high in iron include broccoli, raisins, watermelon, spinach, black-eyed peas, blackstrap molasses, chickpeas, and pinto beans.

Vegetarians need to add vitamin B_{12} to their diet. Some cereals, such as Grape-Nuts, and fortified soymilks have vitamin B_{12} (check the label). Red Star T6635 nutritional yeast flakes (Vegetarian Support Formula) also supply vitamin B_{12}.

Getting Fit with Your Favorite Exercises

Look at your body and decide which areas need the most work. In addition to reducing the body's fat reserves and building energy, exercise keeps you fit, relaxes you, and helps you to manage stress better. The key ingredients for establishing a successful exercise regimen are discipline and consistency. Begin by finding a convenient place where you can work out. Try to do at least fifteen to twenty minutes of exercise before you start your day. If you have time before or after school, you could work out on your bedroom floor, on your patio, or in your yard. Make sure you have the tools you'll need, such as hand weights, a fitness mat, and maybe a jump rope or step bench. If you have a break during the day, perhaps you can go to a nearby park, a health club, or a gym. You might be able to do a set of abdominal curls, push-ups, or arm exercises using weights. Whatever form of exercise you choose, remember, you can make it a habit if you always keep it convenient and practical.

Smart *and* Sensible Suggestions for You

If you're just beginning an exercise program, start by walking on a treadmill or outside for fifteen to twenty minutes, three times a week. After you walk, do some light stretches for your back, legs, and hips. Then incorporate some sit-ups. As you get stronger and more comfortable with exercise, add resistance training to the upper and lower body by using light weights. A personal trainer can help you learn how to use the equipment at a gym. Workout videos are also a great way to work out at home. Be consistent, patient, and don't give up.

Don't rush your decision. Do some research and try various methods. There are so many interesting and exciting ways to get and keep a fit body such as: walking, running, stretching, swimming, bicycling, skating, various sports activities, yoga, aerobics, stepping, spinning, and lifting weights. You can work out alone, with a personal trainer, with your best friends, or with a team. Enjoy whichever method you choose, because it could lead to a lifetime of fitness. Do it, and you will win!

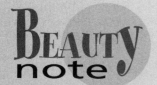

Body Stretch Marks

Body stretch marks around the neck, armpits, stomach, buttocks, and thigh areas, which may appear after weight loss, body shaping, and bodybuilding are often hereditary. If they begin to appear, apply cocoa butter on the areas (several times a day, whenever possible), which often lessens the extent of the discoloration.

All in the Game of Sports

For active teens, diet and nutrition are very important. Many of you are playing competitive high school sports in large numbers and may be preparing to carry this skill into the college women's tournaments in competition. If you are an athlete, you are likely to perspire excessively, and therefore you should shower and shampoo a lot.

Moisturizing dehydrated skin is very important for your overall appearance, as well as conditioning your hair daily. I suggest the following regimen:

- Cleanse
- Tone
- Moisturize
- Apply no foundation
- Use a little waterproof, smear-proof mascara
- Use lip liner pencil to match a sheer lipstick color

If you are physically active, eat a great diet, and follow this regular skincare routine, you'll look and feel fabulous.

Basic Beauty Facts

Dry, cracked elbows, knees, and feet mean you're in need of healing hydration, so quench your skin's thirst by drinking plenty of water, avoiding showers that are too hot, and lathering up with gentle, nondrying soaps. Lock in moisture with ultrarich lotions and oils that condition dry skin.

Rest and Relaxation

One of the most important things you can do as a teenager is to value sleep. If you feel tired and there is an opportunity to nap during the day, take it. This doesn't mean you

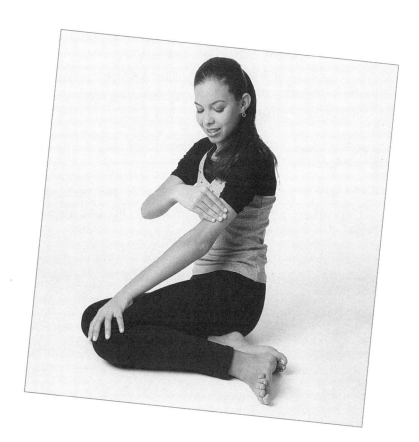

should fall asleep in history class, but that you should take a quick snooze after school, before practice. You naps shouldn't last any longer than an hour and should be planned ahead of time. Falling asleep while trying to do your homework is not a scheduled nap. But if you decide to come home from school, eat a snack, and sleep for forty-five minutes, that will help you control your tiredness.

If you're an athlete who has an important competition coming up in a few days, try to get nine hours of sleep on the nights leading up to the event. If nerves keep you up the night before, at least you will have a few good nights of sleep in the bank. On the night of your game, try to get your homework done in between classes and before the event. That way, instead of coming home exhausted after the game and trying to get your homework done, you'll be able to go straight to bed, which will allow you to get a few more hours of sleep.

In order to get to bed at a reasonable time and fall asleep right away, stay away from the Internet or television before going to bed. Those prebedtime rituals may keep your energy up instead of letting your body wind down. Read instead.

Once the alarm goes off, get up and get moving—especially outside—ASAP. This is a great time to take a walk or do some stretches. Getting into the light right away will help reset your biological clock and let your body know it's time to wake up.

Sleep patterns are developed early in life, so your teen years are a great time to set standards that your body will follow for the rest of your life.

Take Good Care of Yourself

Every day, pause and take time to relax spiritually, physically, and mentally. Spend quiet time releasing any tension that you might have. Breathe silently and deeply and meditate with your eyes shut.

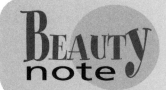

Relaxation Tip
At least twice a year, treat yourself to a professional massage. It will work wonders!

Massage

Massage can be a wonderful therapy. It helps you to relax your muscles, improves circulation, and cleanses the body of toxins. The best time to give yourself a massage is right after you bathe.

Start with your feet, the part of your body that works the hardest. They carry you around all day, and you seldom treat them well. After you bathe, spend a little time applying moisturizing cream to your legs, ankles, and toes. Work the lotion in well between your toes and up and down your legs.

Your arms are next. Apply lotion and firmly work it up and down your arms and shoulders. Continue to massage or knead the arms until you feel all tension released, then work your way up to your shoulders.

Also massage other fleshy areas of your body, such as your abdomen and thighs.

QUIZ

1
Q. What is one of the most important things to develop early in life?
A. Good sleep patterns.

2
Q. What is a vegetarian?
A. Someone who abstains from eating or using animal products, including milk, cheese, or other dairy items, and eggs.

3
Q. How can snacks benefit you?
A. They can be a quick and easy way to refuel your body.

4
Q. What are three different ways to keep your body fit?
A. Walking, running, and stretching.

5
Q. When should you take multivitamins and minerals?
A. They should be used as supplements to a healthy diet and not substitutes for whole foods.

CONCLUSION: THE LAST WORD ON BEAUTY

*B*orn Beautiful is a guide about the beauty of color, a new focus in teenage beauty, and a turning point that acts as an important beacon for teenage girls. While you may recognize that your ancestral roots are in Africa, you have turned homeward to create a culture of fashion and style that is uniquely yours.

Born Beautiful reaffirms and defines beauty for teenagers of color on their own terms. As you read and turned each page, you will have discovered beauty tips to enhance your looks and expand your inner self. You will pull this book from your shelf for quick reference on a new hair color. To enhance your image for that important out-of-town visit, you'll pack your beauty bible in your weekender. You'll share it with your girlfriends or keep it at your bedside to curl up with and plan a new look . . . all with your own distinctive style.

Before I conclude, I want you to consider a few other things that were not mentioned previously. Good looks must be accompanied by facial expressions that reveal warmth and sincere friendliness. Attractive facial expressions add a glow that can make a plain girl stand out in a crowd. A lively smile and sparkling eyes will attract attention, and a face that mirrors a warm and kindly personality has a vivacious quality far more desirable than mere beauty. Let your eyes show joy when you are happy about something and they will delight others as well. Maintain a warm and pleasing voice, whenever possible. Know your grammar, and expose yourself to good speech. Work on your pitch, enunciation, and pronunciation. Just as water keeps your body strong, replenishing it with needed nutrients, so does fresh air keep your lungs strong and help them to breathe more clearly. Good breathing habits make a world of difference in both health and speech. And finally, sit straight and stand tall at all times.

Be proud of yourself. You were Born Beautiful! God bless you!

ACKNOWLEDGMENTS

To my supportive sisters, Beverly and Elizabeth; nieces, Sharmyn, Julie, Darla, Carla, Sherry; and nephew, Troy.

Mentors:

John H. Johnson
Benjamin Wright
Elsie Archer
Dr. Alfred Sloan
Hurley Phillips
Joseph Merriweather
Rose Morgan
John Ledes
Anthony B. Colletti

Carole Hall, editor-in-chief, African American Books, John Wiley & Sons, Inc., for the opportunity and the great idea; Tony Rose, publisher and CEO of Amber Books Publishing for making this book a reality; Yvonne Rose, senior editor of Amber Rose Books Publishing for the flow; Terrie Williams of the Terrie Williams Agency for making the connection; Kimberly Monroe, associate managing editor, and Shelly Perron, copyeditor, for their contributions to producing the book at Wiley; Joan Bowser, Bob Tate, Edward Lewis, Clarence Smith, Susan L. Taylor, Ionia Dunn-Lee, Marcia Ann Gillespie, Mike J. Bramwell, Byron Barnes, Constance White, Brian Basil Daley, Naomi Sims, Alex, Valerie Bennett, Earle Holman, Ashley Hall, John Blassingame, Eddie and Grace Phipps, Edythe Karr, Sybil Gooden, Fred Dillon, Iman, Emmitt Dudley, Gwendolyn Nicholas, Carolyn Florence, Brian Hayes Copeland, Georginia G. Hill, Kelly Rollins, Bernice Coleman, Wanda J. Baskerville, Gloria Pflanz, Darrin Patrick, D'angelo Thompson, Lawrence Burchall, Kelvin Wall, Kendal Aegri, Sherry Bronfman, Audrey Bernard, Barbara Harris, Lu Willard-Stoffman, Evelyn Cunningham, Dr. Gloria E. A. Toote, Esq., Bernice Calvin, Milton Scott, Wentworth Christopher, Bert Emanuel, Sheila Evers, Regina Fleming, Aunt Lois, Walter Greene, Therez Fleetwood, Ronald Lihurd, Alan Price, Roy Hastick, Ruth Sanchez, Emel Lindsay Cross, Jessica Harris, Mary Garthe, Betty Johnson, Bernice Whistleton, Ernest Lee, Joan Murray, Tony, Michael, James Harris, Rudy Townsel, Kathleen Myer Lane, Winston Isaacs, Jacqueline Champagnie, Kowan Choi, Dorothy Pitman Hughes, Ophelia DeVore School of Modeling, Hal Jackson's Talented Teens, Gail and Jimmy Carter, Flora Haynes, Grace Monika, Ananda Lewis, Sharmaine Web, Marvette Britto, LaFrances Singletary, Alnisia Cruz, Jennifer Johnson, Opal Jones, Travis Winkey, and Cynthia Horner.

Amber Books special acknowledgments:

Produced and cowritten by Amber Books Publishing

Tony Rose, publisher and editorial director

Yvonne Rose, senior editor

Samuel P. Peabody, associate publisher

Lisa Liddy, cover and interior design

Alfred Fornay, makeup director

Wayne "Zoom" Summerlin, cover and interior models photographer

Cover models: Genna Young, Jessica Young, Luchia Dickson, Kimberly Butler, and Synchana Elkerson

Nikki Lloyd, cover model and interior model makeup artist

Melanie McKenzie, cover model fashion stylist

Yvonne Rose, cover and interior photo production coordinator

Tony Rose, Yvonne Rose, and Therez Fleetwood, cover photo design

Walik Gorshorn, celebrities backstage photographer

Thanks to our celebrity models: Ananda Lewis, Destiny's Child, Beyoncé, Brandy, Changing Faces, and Kamali Minter

Dwight Carter, step-by-step and interior model photographer

Ashley Hall, step-by-step and interior model makeup artist

Melissa Stenbar, step-by-step model

Alvaro, tools illustrator

Marvin Edwards, home girl photographer

The models: Amilcar Constanza, Elise Tripline, Alessa Price, Martha Ighodaro, Synchana Elkerson, Kimberly Butler, Brittany Johnson, Heather Law, Katurah Miller, Kessiah Basdeo, Vesha Burrell, Luchia Dickson, Jamilah Seabrook, Melissa Stenbar, Rachel Willard, Genna Young, Jessica Young, Kamisha Thompson, La'Toya Johnson, Tasia Henry, Bianco Wideman, Shaquetta Lawrence, Taisha Lawrence, and Tyeka Polanco.

INDEX

acid mantle of skin, 5
acne, 30–31, 34, 45, 47
alcohol, effects on skin of, 6, 8, 10
allergies to makeup, 82–83
antibiotics, 31
astringents, 32, 35, 39, 40, 46

baths, 9, 106
benzoyl peroxide, 30–31
Beyoncé, 68, 69
birthmarks, 48
blackheads and whiteheads, 40, 41, 47–48, 56
bleaching agents, 51
blemishes, 47–48, 56, 57. *See also* breakouts
blow dryers, 139
blushers, 61, 85–90, 98
body piercing, 121, 125–26
braids, 133, 138

Brandy, 129, 130
breakfast, 144
breakouts
acne, 30–31, 34, 45, 47
cleansers and, 25, 47
menstrual periods and, 47
normal-to-combination skin and, 40, 41
oil products and, 9
sensitive skin and, 44
treating, 34, 47–48

caffeine, effects on skin of, 8
calcium, dietary, 150
carotene, 49
Changing Faces, 109, 110
cleansers, choosing, 24–25, 30
cleansers, for eye area, 27–28
cleansing, facial
deep, 28–29, 30, 34, 41

dry skin, 37
normal-to-combination skin, 40, 41
oily skin, 30–35
sensitive skin, 43, 44, 45
color
blusher, 85–86, 87
choosing, 67–71
combining, 69–70
favorites, 83
hair, 134–38
lip, 91–93
nail, 113, 115
quizzes, 70, 100
"rules" about, 66
skin, 49–52, 65, 67
tools, 71–72
combination skin
blushers for, 86
cleansing, 40, 41
climate and, 40, 41, 42
dos and don'ts for, 42
foundation for, 53
regimen for, 39–42

163

combination skin
(continued)
  moisturizing, 27, 40, 41
  testing for, 17, 19
concealers, 57, 58–59, 97
conditioners, hair, 128, 140
cover sticks, 57
curlers, 139

deep-pore cleansing,
  28–29, 30, 34, 41
dermis, 5
Destiny's Child, 26, 27
diet
  effects on skin of, 11–12,
    45, 46, 56
  health and, 144–50
  and nails, 108, 118
  vegetarian, 146–50
discolored skin, 46, 58
drugs, effects on skin
  of, 6
dry skin
  blushers for, 86, 87
  cleansing, 37, 38, 39
  climate and, 7, 16, 38
  dos and don'ts for, 39
  on elbows and knees,
    152
  foundation for, 53
  on hands, 111
  hot baths and, 9
  moisturizing, 9, 26, 27,
    37, 38, 152
  products to avoid, 9, 36,
    39

regimen for, 35–39
sun and, 9
testing for, 17, 19
water and, 5, 10, 13, 35,
  39, 152

electrolysis, 141–49
epidermis, 4–5, 6
epithelial tissue, 5
eruptions. See breakouts
exercise, 10, 151–52, 155
exfoliation, 28, 30, 34, 35,
  38
extensions, hair, 133
eyebrows, 73–76, 78–81,
  89, 90, 98
eyelashes, 74, 75, 84, 98
eyeliners, 74, 75, 81–83,
  98
eye makeup
  allergies to, 82–83
  applying, 77, 80
  for brows, 74, 75, 78, 98
  eyeliner, 74, 75, 81–83,
    98
  mascara, 84, 98
  removing, 34, 38, 41
  shadow, 72, 73–76,
    83–84, 90, 97
eyes, cleansing area
  around, 27–28

face shapes, 88–90,
  128–31
facial expressions, 157
facials, triple-oxygen, 34

foot care, 117–18
foundation, 49–56, 58–59,
  97
fragrances, 102–108, 126

germinating layer of skin, 6

hair
  care of, 128, 138–40
  coloring, 134–38
  facial, 140–41
  quiz, 142
  removing, 140–42
hairpieces, 130, 132–33
hairstyles, 128–34
hairstylists, 131
hand care, 108, 110–11,
  118
hangnails, 114
health
  diet and, 144–50
  quiz, 155
  skin and, 6, 8–12, 45
hemoglobin, 49
henna hair color, 135
henna "tattoos," 119–20,
  121–25, 126

iron, dietary, 150

keloids, 48

Lewis, Ananda, 12, 13
lips
  color for, 91–93
  moisturizing, 32, 38

shape and appearance of, 90–91
sun protection for, 15
lipstick, 93–96, 99

makeup. *See also specific kinds of makeup*
· allergies, 82–83
applying, 96–100
quizzes, 70, 100
tools, 71–72
manicures, 112, 113–14
mascara, 84, 98
masks, facial
for deep-pore cleansing, 28–29
for dry skin, 38, 39
for normal-to-combination skin, 41
for oily skin, 34, 35
for sensitive skin, 44
massage, 154
melanin, 13, 49
menstrual periods and breakouts, 47
milia, 48
Minter, Kamali, 147, 148
moisturizers
climate and, 7, 27
for dry skin, 9, 26, 27, 37, 38, 152
for hair, 128
for lips, 32, 38
for normal-to-combination skin, 40, 41
for oily skin, 26, 32, 33

products to avoid, 9, 36, 39
for sensitive skin, 43, 44
skin type and, 26–27
using, 28
mole removal, 48

nail care, 108–18
normal-to-combination skin, 17, 19, 24, 39–42

oil products, eruptions and, 9
oils in skin, dry skin and, 5, 9
oily skin
blushers for, 86, 87
cleansing, 28
dos and don'ts for, 35
foundation for, 53
moisturizing, 26, 32, 33
regimen for, 30–35
testing for, 17, 18
overeating, effects on skin of, 8

pedicures, 117–18
petroleum jelly, 9, 24, 39
pH factor of skin, 5–6
piercing, body, 121, 125–26
pimples, 45, 47–48. See also breakouts
pomade, 137
powders, face, 59–62, 97
protein, dietary, 149–50

quizzes
Adding Color to Your Face, 100
Essentials about Your Skin, 63
Hairstyles and Hair Care, 142
health and fitness, 155
makeup colors, 70
Those Extra Accents That Define You, 126
What Do You Know About Your Skin? 20–21

rashes, 40
relaxers, hair, 134
resorcinol, 45
rest and relaxation, 152–54
retinoids, 31

scars, 48, 58
scents, 102–108
scrubs, exfoliating, 35
sebaceous oils, dry skin and, 5
sensitive skin
blushers for, 86
cleansing, 43, 44, 45
dos and don'ts for, 45–46
foundation for, 53
moisturizing, 43, 44
regimen for, 42–46
testing for, 17, 19
shampoos, 140

skin. *See also* dry skin; oily
    skin; combination skin;
    sensitive skin
  color, 49–52, 65
  discolored, 46, 58
  don'ts and dos for, 8–12
  flaking of, 4
  functions of, 3
  health and, 6, 8–12, 45
  layers of, 4–6
  oils in, 5, 9
  pH factor of, 5–6
  quizzes, 20–21, 63
  types, 16–19
sleep, 152–54
smoking, effects on skin
    of, 6, 8
snacks, 144, 151
soaps, 24, 39
SPF (sun protection factor),
    15–16

sponges, makeup, 55, 97
sports and skin, 152
straightening combs, 139
stress, effects on skin of, 8,
    31
stretch marks, 152
sun and skin, 5, 9, 13–16
sun protection factor (SPF),
    15–16
sunscreens, 7, 15–16
sweets, 145

tattoos, 119–25, 126
Taylor, Susan, 30, 31, 82,
    121, 126
teeth, 90, 91
toners, 25, 28, 32, 33, 37,
    40, 43
tones, skin, 50, 51, 52, 67
tools, face-coloring, 71–72
triple-oxygen facials, 34

T-zone, 17, 32, 40

undertones, skin, 49, 52,
    67

vegetarian diet, 146–50
vitamin supplements, 12,
    150, 155
voice, quality of, 157

water
  benefits of, 10, 146
  dry skin and, 5, 10, 13,
    35, 39, 152
  filters, 11
  oily skin and, 30, 35
weaves, hair, 132, 138
weight gain, 145
whiteheads, 40, 41, 47, 48,
    56
wrinkles, sun and, 9